Think Like a Nurse
The Caputi Method for Learning Clinical Judgment

Please consider FAIR USE under copyright law:

To use any of the tools and activities in this book,
all users must own their own copy of the book.

Faculty can only use these materials with students
if this book is adopted as a required student textbook.

Thank you,
Linda Caputi

A student textbook that actually teaches a complete, thorough clinical judgment framework.

The Caputi Clinical Judgment Framework is the thinking behind the nursing process and the Next Generation NCLEX®.

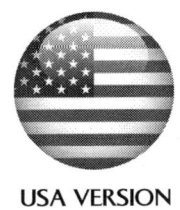

USA VERSION

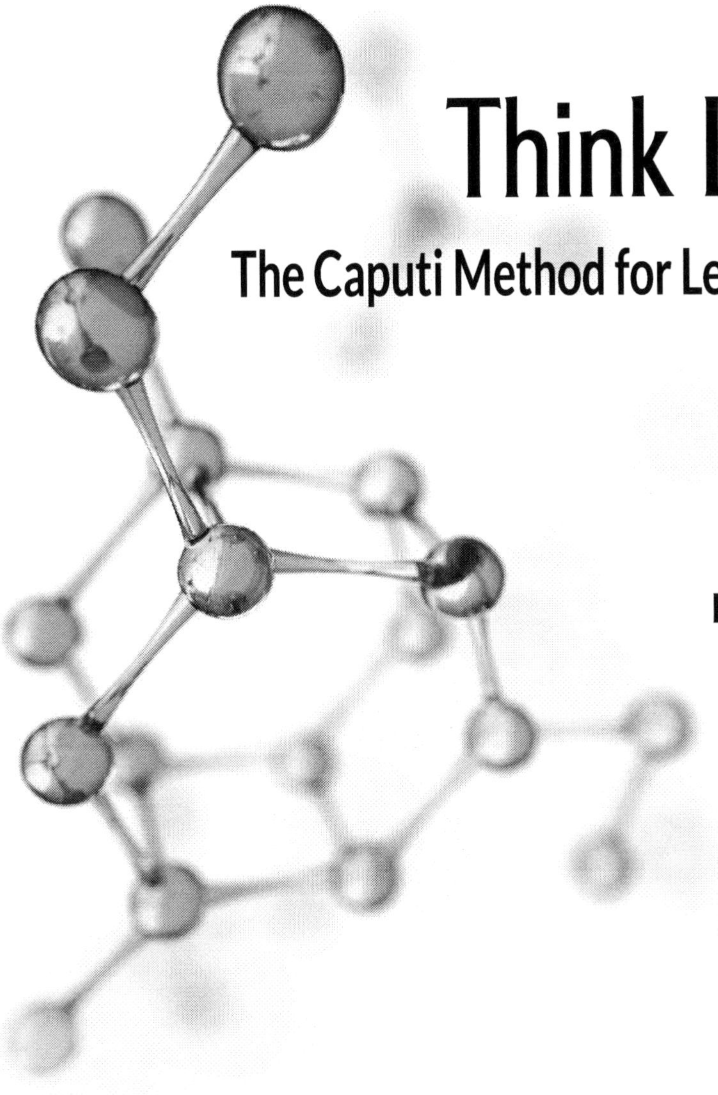

Think Like a Nurse

The Caputi Method for Learning Clinical Judgment

LINDA CAPUTI
RN, MSN, EdD, CNE, ANEF

Think Like a Nurse
The Caputi Method for Learning Clinical Judgment
(USA Version)

© 2022 by Linda Caputi. All rights reserved.
© 2018, 2020 by Linda Caputi. All rights reserved.

All rights reserved. No part of this publication may be reproduced or transmitted in any form or by any means, electronic or mechanical, including photocopy, recording, or any information storage and retrieval system, without permission in writing from the publisher.

Please contact Dr. Linda Caputi at https://LindaCaputi.com for permission to make copies of any part of this work.

Windy City Publishers
www.windycitypublishers.com

Published in the United States of America

ISBN (print):
978-1-953294-20-3

Library of Congress Control Number:
2021925172

Front Cover Image by Egorov Artem/Shutterstock.com
Front Cover Flag Image by pockygallery/Shutterstock.com

WINDY CITY PUBLISHERS
CHICAGO

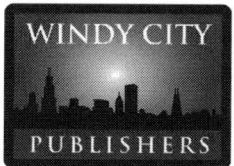

I am honored to dedicate...

... this book to all nursing students
as they develop their passion for nursing
and desire to use clinical judgment
to provide quality, safe patient care
that improves patient outcomes.

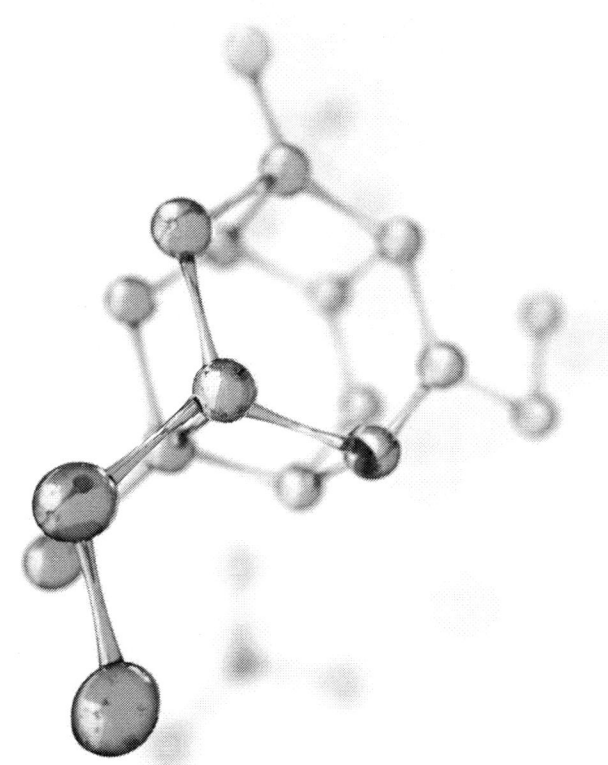

About the Author

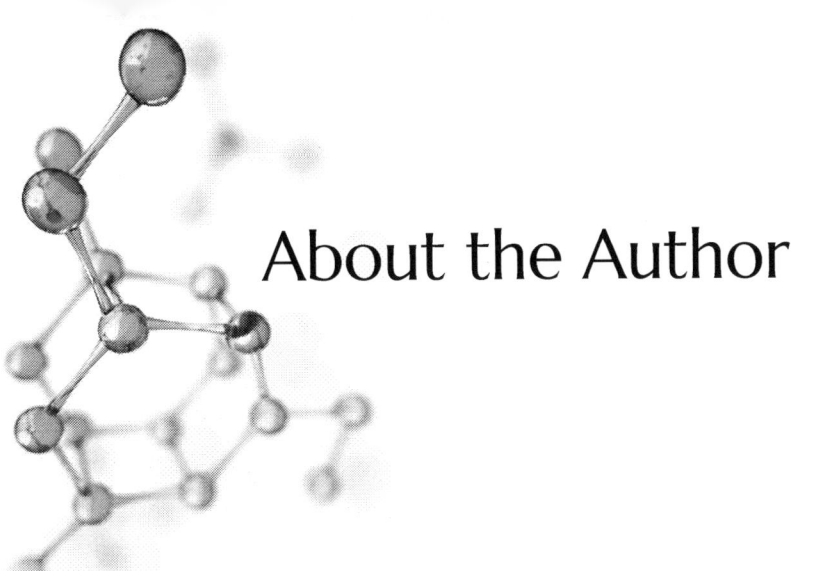

Dr. Linda Caputi
MSN, EdD, CNE, ANEF

DR. CAPUTI IS PROFESSOR EMERITUS, College of DuPage in Illinois. She has taught in LPN, ADN, BSN, and MSN programs. She is President of Linda Caputi, Inc., a nursing education consulting company. Spanning across 30 years, Dr. Caputi has consulted with over a thousand nursing schools on topics related to teaching clinical judgment, revising curriculum, transforming clinical education, test item writing and analysis, student retention, increasing NCLEX pass rates, and numerous other nursing education topics. She has also presented at over 1,000 workshops and nursing education conferences.

Dr. Caputi has won six awards for teaching excellence from Sigma Theta Tau, is included in three years of *Who's Who Among America's Teachers*, was nominated for the Outstanding Teacher Award in 2005 from the National League for Nursing (NLN), and was presented the 2004 Educator of the Year Award from the Organization of Associate Degree Nursing. She is the editor of the second edition (2020) of NLN's *Certified Nurse Educator Review Book* and five other books published by the NLN. She co-authored with Dr. Jean Giddens, *Mastering Concept-based Teaching* (first and second editions). The second edition of her three-volume book *Teaching Nursing: The Art and Science* won the 2010 Top Teaching Tools Award in the print category from the *Journal of Nursing Education*.

Throughout her career, Dr. Caputi has also published numerous book chapters, journal articles, educational software programs, online learning materials, and even board games for nursing students. For ten years Dr. Caputi served as the editor of the Innovation Center, a column in the NLN's journal *Nursing Education Perspectives*. Dr. Caputi is a Certified Nurse Educator, was inducted as a fellow into NLN's Academy of Nursing Education, and has served on the NLN's Board of Governors.

Dr. Caputi's website https://LindaCaputi.com provides more information including an array of teaching resources for faculty.

Authors of Case Studies Used in the Online Course

Donna Badowski & Christie M. Cavallo

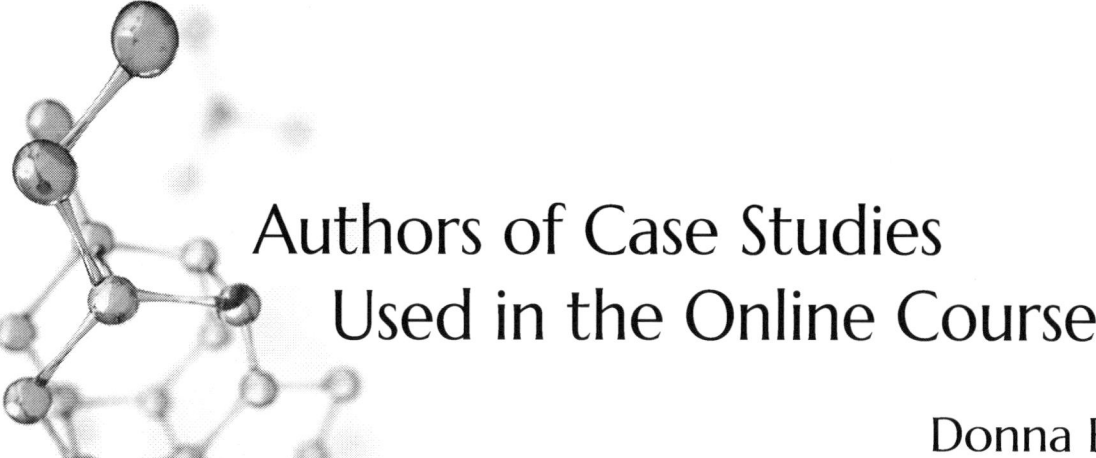

DONNA BADOWSKI ~ DNP, RN, CNE, CHSE *(Author of the Maternal Nursing Case Study)*
Dr. Donna Badowski is an Associate Professor at DePaul University in Chicago. She has been a nurse educator for 17 years and simulationist for 15 years teaching in Practical Nursing, Associate Degree Nursing, Baccalaureate Nursing, and Master Degree programs.

Since 2009, Dr. Badowski has incorporated simulation into nursing education when she began developing simulated clinical days for maternal nursing. In 2011, she received a postgraduate certificate in Simulation Education from Bryan College of Health Sciences. Dr. Badowski is a member of the inaugural cohort of the INACSL Fellows. She has served on the INACSL Research Committee having chaired both the Poster Judging Committee and the Conference Planning Committee. She is currently an INACSL Abstract Reviewer.

Dr. Badowski is an accomplished author with an impressive publishing record in nursing education with both research and innovation articles in peer-reviewed journals to her credit. A large part of Dr. Badowski's publications focus on simulation. Dr. Badowski has conducted and published research on using simulation in nursing education from a variety of perspectives including integrating peer coaching in simulation to improve teamwork and safety, using telehealth simulation for post-licensure nursing students, and conducting national surveys related to various aspects of simulation. Dr. Badowski served as a peer reviewer for the NLN's journal *Nursing Education Perspectives* and is now the editor of the Innovations Center in that publication.

CHRISTIE M. CAVALLO ~ MSN, RN, EdD (c), CNE, CNEcl *(Author of the Adult Health Nursing Case Study)*
Christie M. Cavallo has been a nurse for 28 years and has held various positions in nursing, including bedside patient care in adult health, ICU, cardiac stepdown, PACU, home health, and outpatient surgery. She has spent the past 10 years as a nurse educator in academic nursing programs and currently teaches in the accelerated BSN program at the University of Tennessee Health Science Center in Memphis. Mrs. Cavallo teaches Nursing Concepts 1 and is a simulation champion for the College of Nursing.

Mrs. Cavallo earned a BSN at Delta State University in Cleveland, MS, and a Master in Nursing Education from Walden University in Minneapolis, MN, where she is currently a Doctor of Education candidate. Christie writes a nursing education blog for Wolters Kluwer and serves as a peer reviewer for the ANA Journal *American Nurse Today* and the *Journal for International Nursing*. Christie serves as an exam item reviewer for Elsevier Publishing. Christie is a member of the American Nurses Association, Tennessee Nurse's Association, Tennessee Simulation Alliance, National League for Nursing, and Sigma Theta Tau Honor Society.

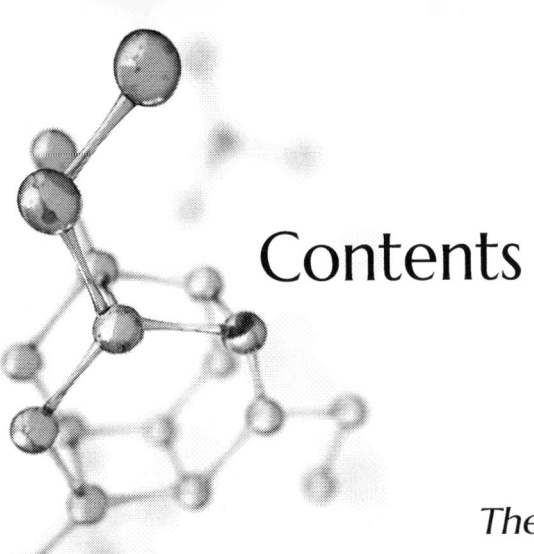

Contents

Think Like a Nurse
The Caputi Method for Learning Clinical Judgment

v	About the Author ~ Dr. Linda Caputi
vii	Authors of Case Studies Used in the Online Course
xiii	Who Should Use This Book
xv	Preface
1	Introduction

SECTION I
Learning To Think with the Caputi Clinical Judgment Framework

5   Chapter 1 ~ Why This Book and Why Learn Clinical Judgment?

23   Chapter 2 ~ The Caputi Method for Learning Clinical Judgment in Nursing

51   Chapter 3 ~ Step 1: Getting the Information (NCLEX® ~ Recognize Cues)
1. Determining Important Information to Collect
2. Scanning the Environment
3. Identifying Signs and Symptoms
4. Assessing Systematically and Comprehensively
5. Ensuring Accurate Information

89   Chapter 4 ~ Step 2: Making Meaning of the Information (NCLEX® ~ Analyze Cues)
1. Clustering Related Information
2. Identifying Assumptions
3. Recognizing Inconsistencies
4. Distinguishing Relevant from Irrelevant Information
5. Judging How Much Ambiguity is Acceptable
6. Comparing and Contrasting
7. Predicting Potential Complications
8. Collaborating with Healthcare Team Members
9. Determining Patient Care Needs/Healthcare Environment Issues

145   Chapter 5 ~ Step 3: Determining Actions to Take (NCLEX® ~ Prioritize Hypotheses & Generate Solutions)
         1. Selecting Interventions
         2. Managing Potential Complications
         3. Setting Priorities

169   Chapter 6 ~ Step 4: Taking Action (NCLEX® ~ Take Actions)
         1. Determining How to Implement the Planned Interventions
         2. Delegating
         3. Communicating
         4. Teaching Others

193   Chapter 7 ~ Step 5: Evaluating Outcomes and Your Thinking (NCLEX® ~ Evaluate Outcomes)
         1. Evaluating Data
         2. Evaluating and Correcting Thinking

SECTION II
Explaining Your Thinking Using the Caputi Clinical Judgment Framework

215   Chapter 8 ~ Advanced Level Cognitive Guidance Tools
         1. What Would You Do Differently?
         2. Worse, Better, or Not Related?
         3. What To Do When?
         4. Effective, Ineffective, or Unrelated?
         5. Determining Nursing Interventions Based on Signs and Symptoms
         6. Planning Safe Care
         7. Pain Assessment
         8. Predicting and Managing Potential Complications
         9. National Patient Safety Goals
         10. Applying Clinical Judgment to Performing Nursing Skills
         11. Relevant Data on Which to Act
         12. What To Do with Data
         13. Planning Patient Care
         14. Comparing and Contrasting Three Patients with the Same Medical Diagnosis
         15. Setting Priorities
         16. Teaching Others
         17. Using Clinical Judgment Competencies to Complete the SBAR Form
         18. Evaluating Data
         19. Evaluating and Correcting Thinking
         20. Safety and Medication Administration
         21. Delegating and Setting Priorities
         22. Calling the Physician or Other Primary Healthcare Provider (PHCP)
         23. Caring for a Patient Post-Procedure
         24. A Quick Look at Planning Patient Care

263   Chapter 9 ~ Clinical Judgment Applied to the Healthcare Setting and Care in the Community

1. Medication Administration from a Systems Perspective
2. Implementing Safety Policies
3. National Patient Safety Goals Applied to a Community Setting
4. Conflict Resolution
5. Analyzing the Electronic Medical Record
6. Creating a Culture of Safety
7. Community Assessment/Windshield Survey

SECTION III

Controlling Your Own Thinking:

Becoming a Self-Directed Thinker by Using the Caputi Clinical Judgment Framework

281   Chapter 10 ~ Putting It All Together

297   References

299   Index

Who Should Use This Book

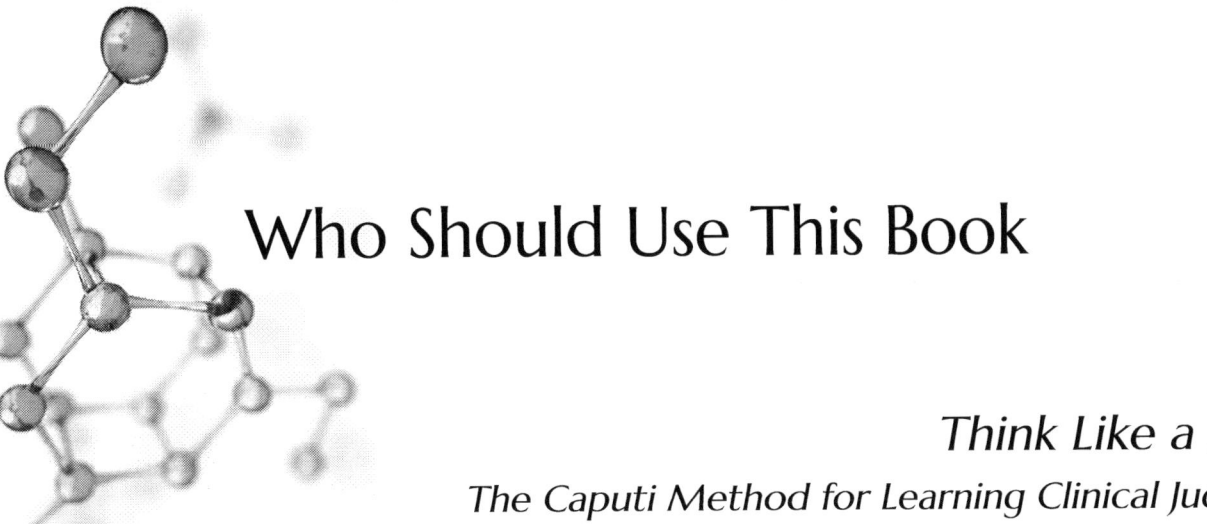

Think Like a Nurse
The Caputi Method for Learning Clinical Judgment

THIS BOOK IS WRITTEN AS a textbook for use in all levels of pre-licensed nursing education: LPN/VN, Associate Degree, Baccalaureate Degree, and entry-level Master's Degree students. It can also be used in all RN to BSN programs as students revisit the process of **developing** clinical judgment, then **applying** it to community health settings and management in the healthcare setting. RN to BSN students can also use this information as they are working with nursing students or orienting new staff in the practice setting. This book is also an excellent resource for nursing professional development practitioners and nurse preceptors as they work with new graduates and new nurse hires to expand their application of thinking as a staff nurse.

Finally, this book is a critical element for all students enrolled in Master in Nursing Education programs. Those being educated as faculty in nursing programs and as nursing professional development practitioners must focus on teaching thinking if we all are to meet the ultimate goal of improved patient outcomes through excellent nursing care.

Please Note:
The tools and activities in this book are for individual use by the person purchasing the book.
Any further use, reproduction, or distribution for use by others is prohibited.

For students to use these tools and activities,
each student must have their own copy of the book.

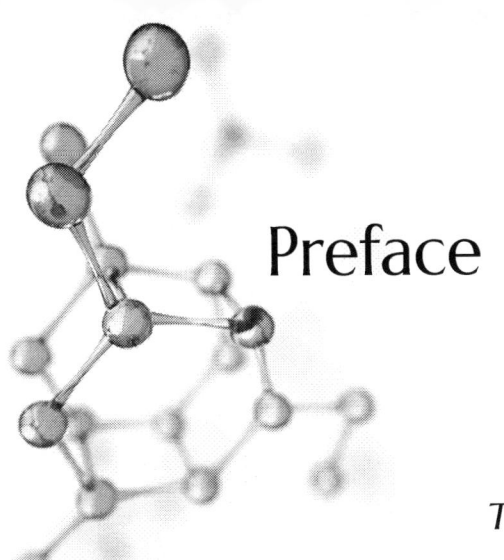

Preface

Think Like a Nurse
The Caputi Method for Learning Clinical Judgment

THE NEW EDITION OF *Think Like a Nurse: A Handbook* actually has a new title, ***Think Like a Nurse: The Caputi Method for Learning Clinical Judgment.*** The name change signifies a maturation of the Caputi Method. The work of developing the Caputi Method has evolved over 20 years and incorporates the full essence of what clinical judgment actually is. The overall goal of this book is to transform an elusive concept—clinical judgment—to an easy-to-learn and understand process applied to nursing. For too long **students** have been unsure what thinking in nursing really is. For too long **faculty** have been led by the misunderstanding that when presented with case scenarios and clinical situations, if students can correctly answer higher cognitive level questions, that means they have learned to "think like a nurse." These students did not learn what clinical judgment actually is; they were just asked questions with the presumption a correct answer meant they could think. This has been a long-standing misconception in nursing education. **Answering a question correctly does not mean the student engaged in thinking to answer the question.** Students actually learning what clinical judgment is and how to use it in nursing is the missing link. A clinical judgment process that uses clinical judgment competencies to connect nursing content to an individual patient situation represents a change in how we teach students to think and a change in how students learn to think. That is what this book is all about.

The changes in this new edition include:

FORMALIZED THE CAPUTI CLINICAL JUDGMENT FRAMEWORK

- This new edition has formalized the Caputi Clinical Judgment Framework.
- The 4-step Tanner Clinical Judgment Model has been replaced with the 5-step Caputi Framework that provides a more complete approach to clinical judgment.
- The term thinking skills and strategies has been replaced with the term clinical judgment competencies.
- The original 19 thinking skills have been retained with the addition of 4 new ones for a total of 23 clinical judgment competencies.
- The entire framework forms the basis for what students need to learn to use the six cognitive processes of the Next Generation NCLEX. The 23 clinical judgment competencies represent the **actual detailed thinking** needed to demonstrate use of the six cognitive processes of the Next Gen NCLEX.

CALL-OUT BOXES

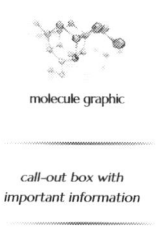

molecule graphic

call-out box with important information

Throughout the book are various call-out boxes to emphasize important thoughts and ideas. Safety and patient-centered care are two major categories of information found in these call-out boxes and are indicated with the *molecule graphic*. These call-out boxes emphasize that clinical judgment supports both safety and patient-centered care. There are additional call-out boxes that emphasize other important information in the text and are indicated with the alternative boxed graphic.

INTRODUCTORY CONTENT

Throughout the book there are many examples of clinical judgment applied to nursing. These examples include nursing knowledge that is new to the beginning student. For this reason, the content mentioned in examples and activities does not represent the full depth and breadth of information on that topic. The intention is to use basic and introductory content so students can focus on learning clinical judgment without getting weighted down with heavy nursing content. Students will learn the nursing content in more depth throughout the nursing program. However, if the book is introduced later in the program, the student should be expected to use the depth and breadth of the material they have learned thus far.

DIVERSITY

The nursing examples provided are very general in nature. They are not meant to represent diverse patient populations, cultures, and ethnic groups. To help students apply the content to diverse populations and situations, they are provided the opportunity to give examples of how they individually use each clinical judgment competency in their own lives. This provides an opportunity for students to demonstrate the use of the clinical judgment competencies in their own world, expressing their personal perspectives when thinking. In class, as students share their personal use of the clinical judgment competencies, they have the opportunity to discover individual, diverse perspectives on the thinking they are learning.

Online Clinical Judgment Course

Starting June, 2022, all schools that adopt *Think Like a Nurse: The Caputi Method for Learning Clinical Judgment* as a required textbook for each student to purchase will have the opportunity for their students to purchase the Online Clinical Judgment Course with Dr. Caputi teaching the content presented in each of the chapters in the book. The online learning discusses the contents of each chapter, includes additional information, and closely links the material to the Next Gen NCLEX. Dr. Caputi applies each of the clinical judgment competencies to unfolding case studies just as students will need to do when taking the Next Gen NCLEX. Using this approach students are not only learning clinical judgment but also learning how to apply clinical judgment in preparation for NCLEX. Students can complete activities for each chapter and upload for faculty review. Faculty can use this Online Clinical Judgment Course as a "hybrid" course for students to learn the material that faculty then apply in class and throughout the nursing courses, as a totally online course, or as homework for a synchronous face-to-face or a synchronous virtual course.

Visit https://LindaCaputi.com for more information.

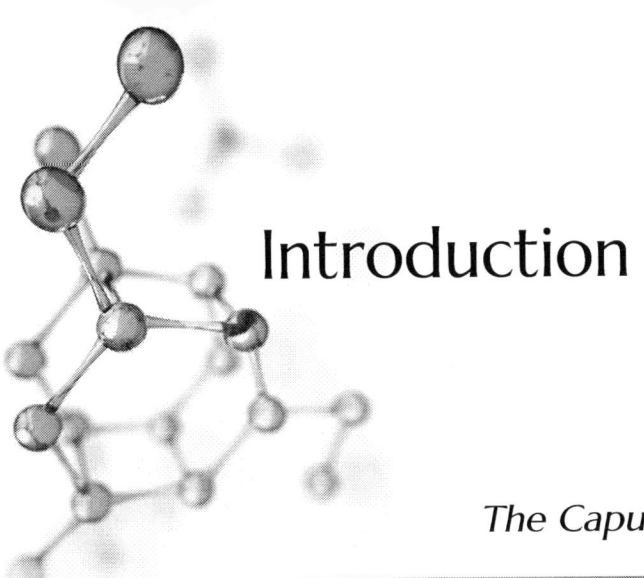

Introduction

Think Like a Nurse
The Caputi Method for Learning Clinical Judgment

THE OVERALL PURPOSE OF THIS book is to teach clinical judgment needed to be a self-directed thinker in nursing. A self-directed thinker is able to determine what thinking is needed in a particular nursing situation without prompts or guidance from another person. Each section of this book focuses on one of three goals that contribute to this overall purpose:

SECTION I

Breaks down clinical judgment into three parts.
All the pieces that make up each of the three parts are taught separately
for a complete understanding of what clinical judgment actually is.

SECTION II

Provides practice working through nursing experiences using
the Caputi Clinical Judgment Framework as a complete entity.

SECTION III

Guides students in self-directed thinking.

The plan is for the student to use this textbook throughout an entire nursing program. During the first term (semester, quarter, whatever type of system a particular school uses) the student works through Section I. During the next several terms of the nursing program, the student continues to use many of the thinking activities from Section I while implementing the learning in Section II. The activities and learning in Section III are accomplished during the final term of the nursing program.

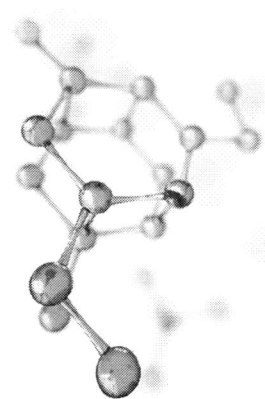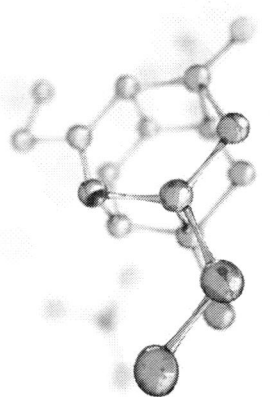

SECTION I

Learning To Think with the Caputi Clinical Judgment Framework
(Chapters 1 - 7)

AS YOU ENGAGE IN DISCUSSIONS with your faculty and preceptors, you will be asked to explain your thinking. You will be expected to **apply thinking** in your explanations. You will also be expected to **apply thinking** to determine answers to additional questions your faculty ask. But how can you apply thinking if you haven't learned what thinking in nursing (clinical judgment) actually is?

Often times if a student has the correct answer to a question or provides explanations with content and rationales that are correct, it is assumed the student **applied clinical judgment**. However, a correct answer does not provide evidence of applying clinical judgment. Merely having the right answer does not mean clinical judgment was actually used to arrive at the answer. It is unsafe to assume students know how to think in nursing without the students:

Merely having the right answer does not mean clinical judgment was actually used to arrive at the answer.

1. Learning what thinking in nursing (clinical judgment) actually is.
2. Being able to explain answers—not just with the content that relates to the answer—but the actual thinking processes (clinical judgment competencies) that were applied to the content, and how the clinical judgment competencies were used in that specific situation.

In the chapters in Section I you will learn the details of the Caputi Clinical Judgment Framework. You will learn the "nitty-gritty" of what thinking in nursing really is and how to engage in that thinking. You will then use this framework of clinical judgment competencies to actually explain the thinking processes you used when faculty ask you to **apply thinking**. Learning the Caputi Clinical Judgment Framework provides a process for you to use throughout nursing school and throughout your nursing career.

In Section II *(Chapters 8 and 9)*~
You will practice explaining your use of clinical judgment by applying what you learned in Section I.

In Section III *(Chapter 10)*~
You will demonstrate how you have become a self-directed thinker.

That is the overall goal of this entire book—helping you to become a self-directed thinker in nursing.

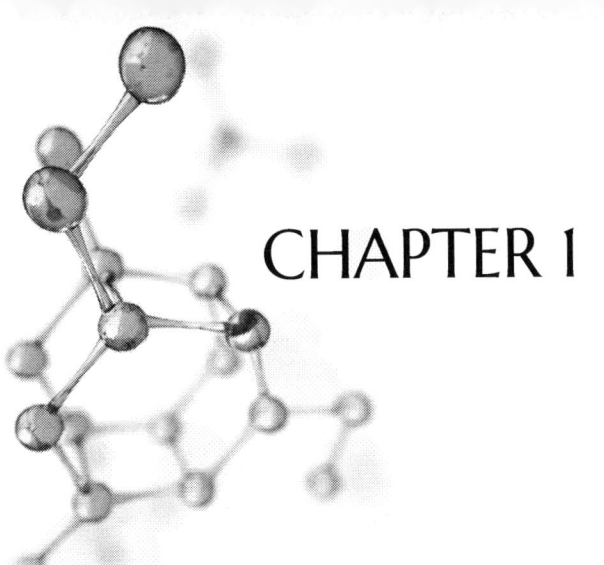

CHAPTER 1

Why This Book and Why Learn Clinical Judgment?

CLINICAL JUDGMENT IS ONE OF the most important topics you will study in your nursing program. Good decision-making by a nurse who is well-versed in clinical judgment is the major factor in keeping patients safe and improving patient outcomes. Ensuring safety and improving care outcomes are goals for each and every patient, population, and community in your care. These goals are not attainable if the nurse does not know how to think; and thinking in nursing requires clinical judgment. This book teaches the clinical judgment you will use to make sound, safe decisions. All patients deserve a nurse who can think.

Good decision-making by a nurse who is well-versed in clinical judgment is the major factor in keeping patients safe and improving patient outcomes.

Critical Thinking Versus Clinical Judgment

Critical thinking, when applied to nursing, is termed "clinical judgment" or, sometimes, "clinical reasoning." There are other terms that may be used, but these two terms are the most common. This text uses the term "clinical judgment." The National Council of State Boards of Nursing defines clinical judgment as:

> Clinical judgment is defined as the observed outcome of critical thinking and decision making. It is an iterative process that uses nursing knowledge to observe and assess presenting situations, identify a prioritized client concern and generate the best possible evidence-based solutions in order to deliver safe client care. (NCSBN, 2019, p. 1)

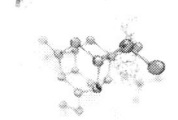

clinical judgment ~ the observed outcome of critical thinking and decision making

This definition of clinical judgment may appear to be somewhat daunting and even a little overwhelming. **This is exactly why this book will be helpful to you!** *Think Like a Nurse: The Caputi Method for Learning Clinical Judgment*

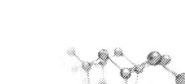

self-directed thinker ~

independent thinkers who can explain their thinking, determine what thinking needs to be employed in a particular situation, then apply their thinking to arrive at a sound decision

breaks down what you need to know so you can learn the pieces of clinical judgment in an easy, understandable way. Then you will use that framework of clinical judgment across your nursing courses as you work through case studies and care for patients in the simulation laboratory and in clinical. That repeated use of the clinical judgment framework prepares you to be a self-directed thinker by the end of your nursing program. Becoming a self-directed thinker (one who knows how to search out the needed information) is necessary to pass the NCLEX and to provide safe, effective patient care as a licensed nurse.

There are a number of reasons to use this book to learn clinical judgment. The reasons include:

1. Preparing for the NCLEX
2. Transforming your everyday thinking to clinical judgment to provide safe patient care and improve patient outcomes
3. Becoming resilient
4. Becoming a self-directed thinker
5. Using situation-based thinking
6. Dealing with unexpected occurrences and reducing errors in the healthcare setting

REASON #1

Preparing for the NCLEX

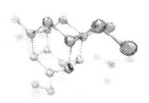

NCSBN ~

the National Council of State Boards of Nursing writes the national licensing exams for both LPN/VNs and RNs

NCLEX ~

the National Council Licensure Examination

The National Council of State Boards of Nursing (NCSBN) is the body that writes the national licensing exams for both Licensed Practical/Vocational Nurses (LPN/VN) and Registered Nurses (RN). To ensure the newly graduated, pre-licensure nursing candidate can use clinical judgment for safe patient care, the NCSBN changed the exam starting in 2023 for both the NCLEX-RN and the NCLEX-PN/VN. The primary change in these new licensing exams is to administer an exam that measures the candidate's ability to engage in clinical judgment at a safe, entry level.

The NCLEX measures the candidate's:

1. Knowledge of nursing content
2. Ability to apply clinical judgment using nursing content to make safe patient care decisions

However, clinical judgment was not directly measured in the pre-2023 version. The new version of these exams is called the Next Generation NCLEX (NGN). The NGN directly measures the candidate's ability to engage in clinical judgment.

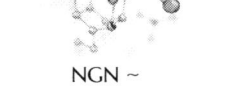

NGN ~
Next Generation NCLEX

When the term "generation" is used as an adjective, it is used to indicate a major change in whatever the word is describing. For example, the Next Generation of cell phones represents a major change in the capabilities of the cell phone. That same use of the word "generation" applies to the name of the NCLEX—the Next "Generation" NCLEX. The Next Generation NCLEX indicates a major change in the licensing exam. **That major change is a very focused evaluation of the new graduate's ability to engage in clinical judgment, or the graduate's ability to think and make safe patient care decisions.**

The NGN Clinical Judgment Measurement Model

How does the NGN measure clinical judgment? There are six cognitive processes measured using the NCLEX Clinical Judgment Measurement Model (NCSBN, 2019):

1. **Recognize Cues**: "Identifying relevant and important information from different sources" (p. 4)

2. **Analyze Cues**: "Organizing and linking the recognized cues to the client's clinical presentation" (p. 4)

3. **Prioritize Hypotheses**: "Evaluating and ranking hypotheses according to priority (urgency, likelihood, risk, difficulty, time, etc.)" (p. 5)

4. **Generate Solutions**: "Identifying expected outcomes and using hypotheses to define a set of interventions for the expected outcomes" (p. 5)

5. **Take Actions**: "Implementing the solution(s) that address the highest priorities" (p. 6)

6. **Evaluate Outcomes**: "Comparing observed outcomes against expected outcomes" (p. 6)

NCLEX
CLINICAL JUDGMENT
MEASUREMENT MODEL

Recognize Cues

Analyze Cues

Prioritize Hypotheses

Generate Solutions

Take Actions

Evaluate Outcomes

The NCLEX uses these cognitive processes to **measure** or **evaluate** the candidate's ability to use clinical judgment. For new nursing students, these six cognitive processes may seem overwhelming.

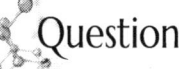

Question

How does a nursing student learn to think using the six cognitive processes measured by the Next Gen NCLEX?

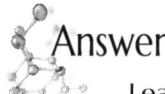

Answer

Learn the Caputi Clinical Judgment Framework presented in this text!

Comparing the NGN Clinical Judgment Measurement Model to the Caputi Clinical Judgment Framework

clinical judgment competencies ~

thinking skills and strategies needed to engage in good decision-making required on the NCLEX

It is important to understand the difference between the NCSBN's Clinical Judgment Measurement Model and the Caputi Clinical Judgment Framework. The NCLEX Clinical Judgment Measurement Model is used to **measure** the test taker's ability to engage in clinical judgment. The Caputi Clinical Judgment Framework is used to **teach** students how to **learn and use** clinical judgment that is measured by the NCLEX. The goal is that when graduates take the NCLEX they have learned to think (use clinical judgment) in the way the NCLEX measures clinical judgment.

This book teaches you all the thinking skills and strategies (which I will call clinical judgment competencies when discussing clinical judgment) you need to engage in good decision-making required on the NCLEX. When you answer questions on the NCLEX you will apply the thinking you learned in this book—thinking that relates to the six processes of the NCLEX's Clinical Judgment Measurement Model.

Table 1.1 demonstrates the way in which this book prepares you to use each of the six cognitive processes measured on the NCLEX. Just learning about the six cognitive processes in the left column is not enough. **Students must learn the thinking behind each step.** The clinical judgment competencies taught in this book provide the building blocks that support the thinking required for each of the six cognitive processes in the NCSBN's Clinical Judgment Measurement Model and tested on the NCLEX. In other words, without learning the specific clinical judgment competencies, it will be very difficult to engage in the clinical judgment required to pass the NCLEX.

TABLE 1.1

How the Caputi Clinical Judgment Framework Supports the Thinking of the NCLEX Clinical Judgment Measurement Model

The Cognitive Processes of the NCLEX NGN Clinical Judgment Measurement Model	Major Steps in the Caputi Clinical Judgment Framework	The Caputi Clinical Judgment Competencies Used with Each of the Six Cognitive Processes of the NGN
1. Recognize Cues	Getting the Information	• Determining important information to collect • Scanning the environment • Identifying signs and symptoms • Assessing systematically and comprehensively • Ensuring accurate information
2. Analyze Cues	Making Meaning of the Information	• Clustering related information • Identifying assumptions • Recognizing inconsistencies • Distinguishing relevant from irrelevant information • Judging how much ambiguity is acceptable • Comparing and contrasting • Predicting potential complications • Collaborating with healthcare team members • Determining patient care needs/healthcare environment issues
3. Prioritize Hypotheses	Determining Actions to Take	• Setting priorities
4. Generate Solutions	Determining Actions to Take	• Selecting interventions • Managing potential complications
5. Take Actions	Taking Action	• Determining how to implement the planned interventions • Delegating • Communicating • Teaching others
6. Evaluate Outcomes	Evaluating Outcomes and Your Thinking	• Evaluating data • Evaluating and correcting thinking

The Caputi Clinical Judgment Competencies listed in the right-hand column of Table 1.1 are what **students absolutely need to learn** to be able to make safe, patient-centered care decisions as tested on the NCLEX. As previously noted, by learning these 23 clinical judgment competencies you are learning the building blocks that support the six cognitive processes of the NCLEX Clinical Judgment Measurement Model. These Clinical Judgment Competencies are **the most important part of learning** clinical judgment. This book provides what you need to learn to think in the way you will be expected to think to pass the NGN.

It is important to know that the Caputi Clinical Judgment Framework taught in this book prepares you for the NGN. ***However***, what is taught in this book also prepares you for the current NCLEX, which is being administered before the NCLEX changes to the NGN in 2023. Additionally, the types of questions currently on the NCLEX will still appear on the NGN. The NGN will be a mix of the current types of NCLEX questions and the Next Gen NCLEX clinical judgment questions.

The Caputi Clinical Judgment Framework prepares you to think at a very high level in a systematic way to make patient care decisions. This prepares you to think—plain and simple. If you learn how to think, then you'll be prepared to pass the NCLEX in any form.

If you learn how to think, then you'll be prepared to pass the NCLEX in any form.

REASON #2

Transforming Your Everyday Thinking into Clinical Judgment for Safe Patient Care and to Improve Patient Outcomes

The purpose of this book is to bring to your awareness the steps you take when solving problems in your everyday life. The fact is, you already know how to think. Once that is brought to your attention, you can become consciously aware of the processes you use to make decisions and the various thinking skills you use every day. These thinking skills are then applied to nursing.

The critical thinking of everyday life and the thinking skills used with critical thinking are applied to nursing. In nursing situations, critical thinking is called clinical judgment and the thinking skills used in everyday life become clinical judgment competencies. See Table 1.2.

TABLE 1.2

Everyday Thinking and Thinking Like a Nurse

	EVERYDAY THINKING	THINKING LIKE A NURSE
Type of Thinking	Critical Thinking	Clinical Judgment
Thinking Processes Used	Critical Thinking Skills and Strategies	Clinical Judgment Competencies

This text helps you become aware of your own problem-solving processes and the thinking you use when making decisions. This thinking is organized in a framework. That framework is the heart of learning to think like a nurse.

You will learn how to apply your everyday thinking to nursing for the purpose of providing safe, quality, patient-centered care; improving patient outcomes; and improving the healthcare environment in which you work. The *Future of Nursing* (IOM, 2011) report reminded us that nurses not only do nursing, but they also improve nursing. Engaging in nursing practice and improving nursing practice both require clinical judgment.

> You will learn how to apply your everyday thinking to nursing for the purpose of providing safe, quality, patient-centered care; improving patient outcomes; and improving the healthcare environment in which you work.

Everyday Thinking Versus Thinking in Nursing

Clinical judgment, the type of thinking nurses use, is **deliberate, skillful, responsible, and thoughtful**. Nurses use a deliberate process for engaging in clinical judgment in their professional roles.

It is important to note that if you were to ask experienced nurses about the deliberate thinking process they use, it is likely most nurses will not be able to explain the step-by-step thinking used that led them to a conclusion. This also may be true if someone asked **you** to explain your step-by-step thinking when working through everyday problems. You have not really thought about how you solve problems; you just do it. You are not consciously aware of the thinking you do, although you have been solving problems for years. As with you, this is the case with most experienced nurses because most nurses in practice are at the expert level of functioning.

> Clinical judgment is deliberate, skillful, responsible, and thoughtful.

Experts use intuitive thinking and no longer delineate or recall each step of the thinking process. Their thinking has become automatic. They control their own thinking (self-directed thinking), but they do so in such a quick fashion that they are not consciously aware of all the steps of thinking they performed. This works for the expert nurse; it does not work for the student learning to be a nurse.

The reason it does not work for nursing students is they do not have the depth of knowledge and the multiple experiences of expert nurses.

Just as you will learn to perform nursing skills, step-by-step, so will you learn to think, step-by-step. The more you use the various clinical judgment competencies, the more automatic using them will become. That is the goal of learning and practicing all the pieces of clinical judgment. Learning clinical judgment does not just "happen on its own," any more than learning to perform a nursing skill "happens on its own." The student must learn the process, understand all the steps of the process, and use the process over and over to become a skillful thinker.

The purpose of this book is to help you become aware of the fact that you already know how to think, apply the thinking you already use to what you need to learn about clinical judgment in nursing, and use that clinical judgment as a nurse. The book provides a framework and a language for you to use to learn clinical judgment and then communicate your thinking (clinical judgment) to others.

REASON #3

Becoming Resilient

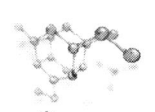

resilience ~

the capacity to accurately perceive and respond well to stressful situations

Another reason to learn the Caputi Method for Learning Clinical Judgment is to help you become resilient in your role as a nurse. So what does learning clinical judgment have to do with becoming resilient, and what does being resilient mean? Sieg (2020) defines resilience as "the capacity to accurately perceive and respond well to stressful situations" (para. 2).

The healthcare environment can, at times, be a very stressful place. Healthcare settings are very dynamic environments; circumstances can change often and very quickly. The unexpected can happen without much warning. The nurse must be ready to respond immediately. Responding immediately means staying calm and having a process for thinking through problems to focus your thinking during stressful situations. Self-directed thinkers who are in control of their thinking by using the clinical judgment framework in this book will be more resilient than nurses who are not able to control their own thinking. Being resilient and in control of your thinking is the first step to responding well to stressful situations.

Focusing your thinking using the Caputi Clinical Judgment Framework requires you to be mindfully engaged in your thinking. Being mindful is mandatory when providing care focused on the individual patient. Sheridan (2016) defines mindfulness as "the ability to be fully present and attentive in the moment" (p. 29). To be fully present in the moment has become more difficult in today's world. People are often interrupted by the ding of their cell phones indicating a new email, text, or voicemail. Even though it appears the person with the phone alert continues to speak, that person is likely thinking about who the message is from or what it might say. The mind is constantly being pulled in other directions. It may be easy to remain mindful for a few seconds; the key is to **stay** mindful. Staying mindful has been shown to lower stress, protect health, and lift mood (Hanson, 2018).

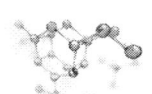

mindfulness ~

the ability to focus and be fully present in the moment

It is sometimes difficult to stay mindful in stressful situations which may occur during patient care. However, staying mindful is critical for safe patient care. Practicing mindfulness builds resilience. Using the Caputi Clinical Judgment Framework in this book helps guide you with a thinking process that keeps your attention on the patient and the situation at hand.

Nurses must be mindful, present, and engaged with the patient. Using the Caputi Clinical Judgment Framework working through the clinical judgment competencies provides a way to stay grounded by using a process to work through to ensure clinical judgment is skillfully implemented.

The framework serves as a guide that gets you back on track with your thinking if you are momentary distracted or interrupted—it helps you focus on what you are doing and to cope better with distractions. This ability to focus (mindfulness) is basic to becoming resilient, a state in which you will be able to accurately perceive and respond well to stressful situations by using the clinical judgment competencies you learn in this textbook.

REASON #4

Becoming a Self-Directed Thinker

Self-directed thinkers are independent thinkers who can explain their thinking, determine what thinking needs to be employed in a particular situation, then apply their thinking to arrive at a sound decision. A major goal of this book is to help you become a self-directed thinker. This book provides what you need to "internalize" a thinking process, but you will need to put forth the effort and motivation to learn and use the process taught. Basically, learning requires time and effort. Learning takes effort (Brown, et al, 2014).

This book provides lots of practice activities. It is important for you to use these activities, gather information, engage in thinking, review your work, present your work to your teacher/preceptor, and request feedback.

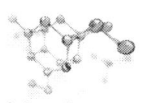

debriefing ~
a critical conversation between you and your teacher/preceptor which provides a critique about your thinking that reinforces correct thinking and clarifies misconceptions

Feedback is also known as debriefing. Debriefing is a critical conversation between you and your teacher/preceptor which provides a critique about your thinking. This debriefing feedback reinforces your correct thinking and clarifies any misconceptions you may have. Debriefing is critical to your learning. These practice activities with feedback are mandatory to learn clinical judgment. It is important to realize that just reading this book, even if you read it over and over, does not mean you know how to think. You must actually engage in the thinking activities to:

1. **Learn what you still need to learn about thinking even if you believe you understand what you are reading in the book.**
   Learning to think is an "inside job" that takes place only when you use clinical judgment in actual or simulated patient situations. Compare learning to think to learning a nursing psychomotor skill, such as hanging an intravenous (IV) solution for infusion. You can read about that skill over and over, but you do not know if you can actually perform that skill if you never hang an IV container of fluids. Additionally, the more IV infusions you administer, the more skillful you become. This same explanation applies to learning thinking skills.

   If you do not complete the activities in this book that guide your thinking you will not know if you can actually engage in the thinking required of a nurse. You will need to keep this textbook throughout your nursing program because it includes activities you will use in the later terms of your program that require you to engage in higher levels of thinking.

2. **Solidify the process into your long-term memory.**
   The more you engage in thinking, the deeper that learning becomes as it moves into your long-term memory. Learning that is stored in your long-term memory is then available for recall and application at a later time. As you move through your nursing program you will retrieve what you learned earlier in the nursing program about the clinical judgment competencies. As you enroll in nursing courses throughout the program and provide care for more complex patients, you will constantly pull forward (retrieve) all that you learn in the early part of this book about using the clinical judgment competencies. This constant retrieval and use of the clinical judgment competencies further solidifies your learning, resulting in deeper learning, which is more easily retrieved when needed (Brown, et al, 2014).

Nilson (2013) conducted a literature search about the benefits of self-directed thinking and found learning in this manner, using deliberate practice, enhances:

1. Student performance/achievement
2. The amount and depth of student thinking
3. Students' conscious focus on their learning (mindfulness)
4. The development of reflective and responsible professional behavior

Many students, and even graduates in their first nursing position, are not aware of the thinking processes they use. Becoming a self-directed thinker means you are consciously aware of your thinking. Your thinking is a planned process not a "hit or miss" process. Clinical judgment is not magical or mysterious, although when talking with an expert it may appear to be. On many occasions when I hear an expert speak, I wonder how that person was able to use the knowledge of the field and arrive at such as conclusion. I am truly impressed. I often think that person must possess some superhuman power. However, the reality is, that person was able to **engage in thinking at a very high level** to arrive at that conclusion. That high-level thinking was achieved by first learning how to think and practice thinking on many occasions and in a variety of contexts (situations). In other words, **deliberate practice with contextual (situation-based) thinking**.

High-level thinking is achieved by first learning how to think and practice thinking on many occasions and in a variety of contexts.

Deliberate Practice

It is one thing to learn about clinical judgment; another to use clinical judgment. Early research on the way nurses think focused on understanding clinical judgment but not specifically on using clinical judgment (Capelletti, et al, 2014). Nursing education must first teach students about what clinical judgment is so students have an understanding of all the thinking processes used with the clinical judgment competencies. Students must then put that understanding into action and use clinical judgment. Asking students to "apply thinking to this situation" is vague and does not engage the learner in the actual clinical judgment process. Applying thinking must be deliberate; meaning a clear method is used. This clear, understandable method is the framework taught in this text. Students must deliberately engage in using each of the clinical judgment competencies to guide their thinking.

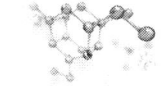

deliberate practice ~

using a clear method of thinking to develop clinical judgment

Deliberate practice using what you learn and understand about clinical judgment provides the opportunity to put your learning into action. Nursing school is not only about learning nursing content and nursing skills, it is about **using and putting into action** what you are learning. Taking action is what nursing is all about. Nurses apply clinical judgment, using nursing knowledge, to take action and provide safe patient care. All nursing actions are based on good decisions.

Deliberate practice is the beginning point for achieving expert performance.

It is not easy work. Deliberate practice is hard work that requires repetition, over and over.

The reward of better patient outcomes is worth the effort.

Deliberate practice is the beginning point for achieving expert performance (Nilson, 2013). The path to expert thinking requires many instances of deliberate practice, breaking down all the elements of clinical judgment using the Caputi Clinical Judgment Competencies that are used to reach sound decisions. As you engage in deliberate practice you will constantly reflect on the thinking you used, identify what went right, identify any errors, correct the errors, then use what you learned for the next deliberate practice session. The activities in this book provide a means for the deliberate practice you need to unpack thinking, learn all the clinical judgment competencies, use the clinical judgment competencies, and then reflect on your thinking to learn from any mistakes.

Self-directed thinkers engage in self-assessment. Self-assessment is critical to grow and mature as a thinker. Self-assessment requires you to be responsible for learning how to think and to grow as a thinker. This is known as having an "internal locus of control." The location of the control for learning lies within you. Your teachers and preceptors are important sources of feedback, but the learner must be internally motivated to learn.

Your teachers or preceptors are part of this process. They can help you reflect on your thinking to identify and correct your errors in thinking and provide guidance. This reflection is a critical part of the process. We learn by experience—not necessarily because of the experience, but by reflecting on the experience (Cannon & Boswell, 2016). This method works for learners new to nursing as well as experienced nurses.

Deliberate practice is not easy work. Deliberate practice is hard work that requires repetition, over and over. This repetition is mentally demanding and can be emotionally draining, but it is necessary. The reward of better patient outcomes is worth the effort. Again, compare learning to think to the process for learning a psychomotor skill. Repeated practice is required to perfect the skill. When caring for patients, students request to perform as many psychomotor skills as possible because they realize the more they perform a skill the better they will become at performing that skill.

This truth also applies to learning to be a good thinker. You must have time to describe your thinking, practice thinking, and demonstrate thinking before being assessed on how well you've learned clinical judgment. With deliberate practice, you will demonstrate connections among many pieces of information and discover solutions to problems by applying clinical judgment competencies to nursing. You will do this all within a specific patient context or situation, explaining how your decisions may vary depending on the individual patient. Clinical judgment is important to transforming the nursing information you are learning to useable knowledge, **not just learning information but knowing how to use the information to make the best possible decisions**. Deliberate practice provides opportunities to become an excellent thinker in nursing.

It is critical to point out the major difference between learning and perfecting a psychomotor skill and learning and perfecting clinical judgment. A psychomotor skill is one discrete task. Learning clinical judgment is much more complex, with many variables and factors that many times may not be obvious to the nurse. However, learning to think like a nurse takes time, but is possible and should start on the first day of your first nursing course.

REASON #5

Using Situation-Based Thinking

A major component of critical thinking in everyday life and clinical judgment in nursing is the context in which the situation is occurring. Making a decision that is based on the situation in which it is occurring is called **situation-based thinking**. Situation-based thinking differs from rule-based thinking. Rule-based thinking means you apply a specific rule to all situations regardless of context. In situation-based thinking, how you apply a rule depends on the situation. What is okay in one situation may not be okay in another. You will learn many normal values, guidelines, and general information about nursing practice and patient care. But just as you consider the context of the situation when making a decision in your everyday life, you will consider the context in which the nursing situation occurs.

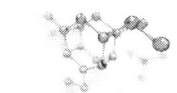

situation-based thinking ~

making a decision that is based on the situation in which it is occurring

Let's look at an example from everyday life. Teens typically have a curfew by which time they need to be home. A curfew time for a teen may be 11 p.m. on Friday and Saturday evenings. On a particular Saturday evening, the teen does not arrive home until 1 a.m. on Sunday. Her parents greet her at the door, say good-night, and retire to bed, as does the teen. There are no problems or issues with the 1 a.m. time. Looking at the situation by simply applying the rule, one would likely conclude the parents must not have been aware of the time. But they were. The difference is that on this evening there was a special dance at the school that did not end until 12:30 a.m. Therefore, the rule was changed for this evening. In this situation the teen returned home on time. Not knowing the context of this situation, it might appear the parents did not act responsibly; however, considering the context in which the situation occurred, the parent behavior is acceptable.

This is a very simple example but demonstrates the importance of considering the context of the situation. This is an important consideration when making decisions in nursing practice and is an overall guideline nurses use in all decision making—**consider the context and engage in situation-based thinking**. Learning clinical judgment as taught in this book will move you beyond using the same rules in every situation (rule-based thinking) to applying the rules in the manner appropriate for the individual patient situation (situation-based thinking).

REASON #6

Dealing With Unexpected Occurrences and Reducing Errors in the Healthcare Setting

Patients often display signs and symptoms, also known as clinical manifestations, that indicate their condition is worsening. The nursing goal is to recognize these manifestations and immediately intervene. Unfortunately, that does not always happen and the warning signs of impending deterioration are not recognized and treated (Purling & King, 2012). Patients can experience acute deterioration in their condition leading to longer hospital stays, unnecessary suffering, and even death. Healthcare agencies need "excellent nurses steeped in the understanding of problem solving" (Kavanagh & Szweda, 2017, p. 57).

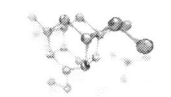

failure to rescue ~

when a patient dies due to complications that were not managed or prevented

Fortunately, most patients for whom you will care will follow a typical path to recovery. The care they require is predictable and manageable by the well-informed nurse. However, you may care for patients who experience an unexpected occurrence, complication, or a pre-existing condition that complicates their recovery. Even the patient who appears to be recovering well can experience a sudden change in their condition. The nurse must be prepared to recognize early, and often subtle, signs of an **unexpected** change in the patient's condition so interventions can be implemented. If interventions are not implemented, the patient may continue to deteriorate. If the patient dies because of complications that were not managed or prevented, this is known as "failure to rescue." The patient died unnecessarily; the death could have been prevented (Odell, 2015). The ability to engage in early recognition of subtle changes in a patient's condition is enhanced and supported by good thinking using clinical judgment.

An additional issue that contributes to poor patient outcomes is the unfortunate reality of errors. Many patients become very ill and even die because of errors made by healthcare personnel (Makary & Daniel, 2016). These errors are often the result of poor thinking processes. Muntean (2012) reported that up to 65% of errors made by nurses that led to negative outcomes could have been prevented if nurses would have made better decisions.

This reality of adverse events and preventable errors in health care is addressed early in this book not to frighten you, but rather to impress upon you why learning clinical judgment is equally important to learning nursing knowledge/content and psychomotor skills. Students often desire to spend their time in class, in laboratory sessions, and in the clinical environment engaging in nursing tasks and may not appreciate the importance of spending time learning and applying clinical judgment. Since students cannot "see" the nurse think, they may not realize just how much thinking the nurse actually does to engage in safe patient care. This lack of ability to visualize the nurse thinking further supports the importance of students repeatedly using all the clinical judgment competencies and working through the activities in this book. Using clinical judgment must start in your initial nursing course and continue throughout all courses of your nursing program. The goal is for your use of clinical judgment to become automatic so that preventable errors are avoided.

Using clinical judgment must start in your initial nursing course and continue throughout all courses of your nursing program.

Factors that Influence the Nurse's Ability to Use Clinical Judgment

At this point it may be helpful to list characteristics or factors that affect your use of clinical judgment.

1. You already know how to think. What you already know how to do will be applied to nursing.

2. Nursing students and nurses think the way they were taught to think.

3. Before students can be asked to "use thinking" they must first learn what thinking is and how thinking is applied in nursing—in the form of clinical judgment.

4. Reflection on decisions made is important to improve thinking. People do not learn by experience alone, but by reflecting on and thinking about their experiences.

5. Sound clinical judgment requires knowledge of the patient and the patient's situation which is also known as situation-based thinking—applying thinking to the specific patient or healthcare situation.

6. Clinical decisions are dependent on the healthcare setting in which they occur (Cappelletti, et al., 2014). This is another aspect of situation-based thinking.

7. Clinical judgment is more influenced by the ability of the nurse to think about a situation than by the objective information related to the situation. That is, the nurse must be able to determine what information is meaningful and how to use that information to make a decision (Tanner, 2006).

8. Nurses must be information seekers.

9. Educational strategies that teach clinical judgment and engage students in using clinical judgment are necessary to learning to think like a nurse.

10. Effective clinical decision making (using clinical judgment) is necessary for positive patient outcomes (Cappelletti, et al., 2014; Tyo & McCurry, 2019).

11. Nurses use self-directed thinking when making decisions.

12. Using specific clinical judgment competencies organized in a framework keeps the nurse focused. Focused thinking is a characteristic of mindfulness; mindfulness contributes to resiliency. As a resilient nurse you are able to accurately perceive (read and understand) a situation, stay calm, remain in control of your thinking, and respond well in stressful situations.

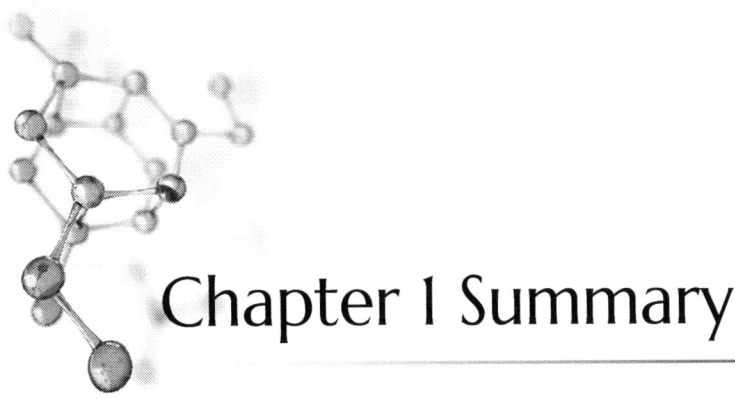

Chapter 1 Summary

The purpose of this book is to offer an evidence-based method for learning clinical judgment in nursing because what—and how—you learn about clinical judgment influences what you bring to patient care. A basic assumption of this book is that the thinking of clinical judgment can be explained and taught. Most nursing students know how to engage in critical thinking in their everyday lives. The issue is they may not realize that the type of thinking they are using to solve everyday problems is actually the same thinking that supports clinical judgment in nursing.

This book presents examples of thinking from everyday life to provide evidence of thinking you currently use. It then teaches how to apply that type of thinking to nursing situations, both when working with patients and when handling situations arising in the healthcare environment. This method connects your everyday way of thinking to a new application of that thinking to demonstrate that thinking in nursing uses the same thinking you may already possess, but that thinking is used within a nursing context. Everyday thinking (critical thinking) applied to nursing becomes clinical judgment. Becoming aware of your everyday thinking is the first step to learning clinical judgment. This awareness demonstrates you are already on your path to learning clinical judgment!

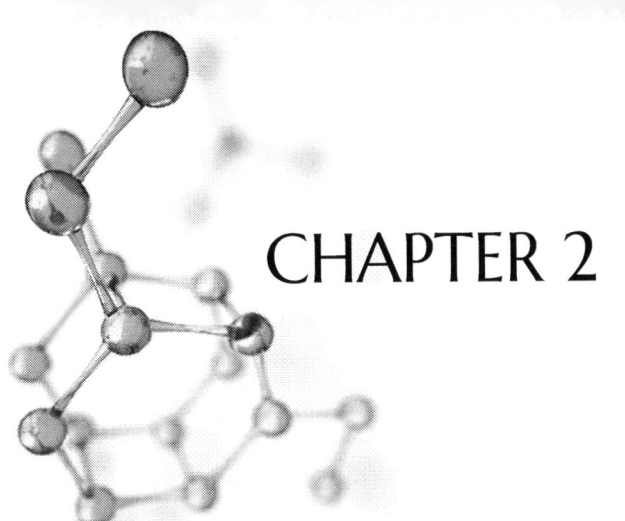

CHAPTER 2

The Caputi Method for Learning Clinical Judgment in Nursing

STUDENTS WANT TO BE NURSES. They see what nurses do and hear what nurses say about the patient's condition and how to care for patients from the medical model perspective. They want to perform as many nursing psychomotor skills as possible. Students cannot "see" nurses think nor do they hear how nurses think. Students may be unaware of the complex thinking that underlies what nurses do. Nurses who are expert in their practice may not be able to describe their thinking, at least not in detailed steps using words that describe a detailed thinking process. Expert nurses work intuitively. Nurses easily know what to do without having explicit instructions about how to do it. They do not consciously work through a thinking process but rather act in a quick, direct manner. Nurses can work in this manner because they are so expert in what they do they no longer work in a step-by-step manner to think about how to do it.

> *Expert nurses work intuitively, and easily know what to do without having explicit instructions about how to do it.*

Think of something you have done for years. Perhaps you have been driving a car for a long period of time. Very quickly explain all you do when you approach a car until you arrive at your destination. You likely cannot explain every decision you made without putting forth a lot of effort to recall what you actually did. In practice, you walk to the car and drive to your destination. You intuitively make dozens of little decisions without giving any of them conscious thought. For example, you quickly start the car, put it in gear, put on turn signals, stop at intersections, know who goes first when another car arrives at that intersection at the same time you do. These are only some of the actions that required thinking that you engaged in but did so intuitively, rather than in a conscious, deliberate manner. This is how experienced nurses work throughout the day.

> *In all aspects of life, not just in nursing, skill in thinking is basic to making quality decisions.*

In all aspects of life, not just in nursing, skill in thinking is basic to making quality decisions. The issue is that thinking, if left to itself, is often not good at all but biased, uniformed, and likely distorted (Paul & Elder, 2020). Unstructured thinking leads to poor decisions, and in nursing, poor decisions can lead to poor patient outcomes. Clinical judgment requires mindful use of thinking processes. That is, clinical judgment should be self-directed and self-corrective. Nurses direct their own thinking. There is no one in the nurse's work environment who is instructing the nurse on how to think. Thinking is an internal process conducted by the individual nurse. Clinical judgment should be self-correcting; that is, the nurse reflects on the thinking to determine whether the thinking was effective and properly used. Good clinical judgment results in the nurse being able to:

> *Clinical judgment requires mindful use of thinking processes, meaning it should be self-directed and self-corrective.*

- Formulate clear and precise questions about the patient to ensure all necessary information is collected and used.
- Gather and analyze relevant information to determine actions to take.
- Ensure accuracy of information collected and how that information is used.
- Skillfully use the information to determine what to do.
- Determine whether the thinking was accurate or if changes in thinking are needed.

To mature as a thinker who is able to use clinical judgment for safe patient care requires a lot of practice (Paul & Elder, 2020). Therefore, once the thinking framework for clinical judgment presented in this book is learned, the thinking processes must be consistently used to ensure the learner moves from a beginner to an advanced thinker prior to graduating from the nursing program. This important aspect of learning clinical judgment was covered in Chapter 1 under the discussion of deliberate practice in the section on "Becoming a Self-Directed Thinker."

Nurses think through, and solve, dozens of problems every day. Many of the problems solved relate to patient care. However, many other problems nurses solve relate to the healthcare environment, interactions with other healthcare providers, constant interruptions, and a host of other issues. Because students cannot see the mental processes in which nurses constantly engage throughout the day, they may not understand the importance of how complicated these thinking processes can be.

This book and the Caputi Clinical Judgment Framework help you uncover and unpack the thinking processes nurses use. This book presents a systematic, formalized method for learning clinical judgment in nursing and how to use that method across the entire nursing curriculum including in the classroom, the nursing laboratories, and the clinical environment.

> *The Caputi Clinical Judgment Framework provides a detailed method for thinking with simple language you can use to communicate your thinking to others.*

Nurse thinking must be unpacked and made clear through specific language that is deliberately taught and used if it is to be valued (Rubenfeld & Scheffer, 2015). Without formal education concerning thinking processes used in clinical judgment, students often struggle to explain their thinking because they have not learned the language of clinical judgment. The Caputi Clinical Judgment Framework provides a detailed method for thinking with simple language you can use to communicate your thinking to others. You may be asked by your teacher to use clinical judgment or to explain your thinking. The language of the Caputi Clinical Judgment Framework makes answering questions and explaining your thinking easier and more precise.

The Three Components of Clinical Judgment

Unpacking clinical judgment begins with identifying its components; that is, what are the parts of the bigger concept of clinical judgment. The Caputi Clinical Judgment Framework (Caputi, 2016, 2020) was formally developed in 2011 after decades of studying the literature on thinking in nursing and applying that research to teach students to think like a nurse. This framework presents a method for learning clinical judgment using specific language that unpacks thinking. Students use this language as they solve problems and make decisions in all nursing environments. The three components of the Caputi Clinical Judgment Framework are:

1. Novice to Expert Theory (Benner, 2001)
2. Steps in Clinical Judgment
3. Clinical Judgment Competencies

These three components overlap to provide a structure for learning clinical judgment in nursing. Figure 2.1 visually connects these three overlapping components that are all part of the bigger process of clinical judgment.

FIGURE 2.1

The Three Components of Clinical Judgment

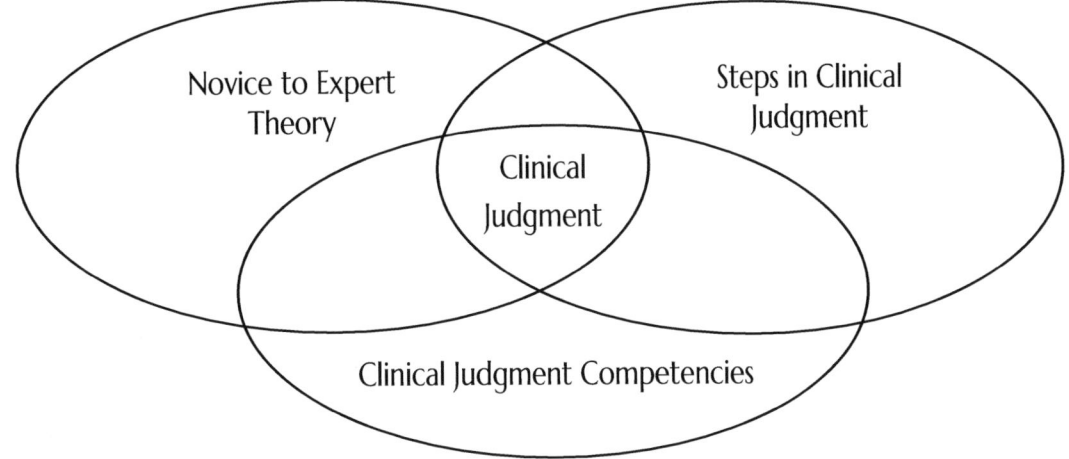

COMPONENT #1

NOVICE TO EXPERT THEORY

The classic theory of novice to expert in nursing (Benner, 2001) describes the stages of cognitive (thinking) development, or skill acquisition, a nurse experiences while moving from a novice to an expert in nursing practice. This theory describes five stages. Learning and using the thinking presented in this book helps nursing students accomplish the first two stages (novice and advanced beginner) while enrolled in a nursing program.

Upon entry to a nursing program the student is considered a Novice. The student arrives with no experience in nursing. Although the student may have worked in another healthcare position, the student has no experience working within the scope of practice at the educational level of the nursing program in which the student is enrolled. For example, if a student enrolled in a Registered Nursing (RN) program is a Licensed Practical/Vocational Nurse (LPN/VN), that student has experience as an LPN/VN but not as an RN. Therefore, the student is a novice in the role of an RN.

When teaching novice nurses, nursing content is broken down into simple, out-of-context terms, so the student can readily understand what is being taught. As a novice, the student learns specific rules to follow and applies these rules to all situations, regardless of context. That is, the student's nursing practice is rule-based. An example of a rule is, "the normal adult blood pressure is less than 120/80 but not so low that the patient is experiencing symptoms such as dizziness." A novice might expect all adults to have a blood pressure somewhat less than 120/80. The novice has not yet learned to handle exceptions to this rule.

At this beginning level, many nursing faculty share with students that nursing is not black or white, but grey. So, what does grey mean? Grey means, "it depends." The "it depends" answer requires situational (contextual) thinking, not rule-based thinking. That is, how the nurse uses the rules that are learned depends on the context of the individual patient situation. For example, the nurse compares a patient's blood pressure of 150/90 to the rule that a normal blood pressure is around 120/80, as described above. Should the nurse take action based on the much higher blood pressure reading of 150/90? Thinking situationally, a much higher or lower blood pressure may be acceptable **depending on the individual patient situation**. This is the "it depends" or "grey" part of nurse thinking.

The "it depends" thinking requires consideration of the individual patient's situation. Students may hear faculty say they must "look at the bigger picture." This is what is meant by that request. Looking at the bigger picture means

How the nurse uses the rules that are learned depends on the context of the individual patient situation.

looking at the entire patient situation to determine how to apply the rules learned. This way of thinking is at the heart of patient-centered care: determining nursing actions based on the collected patient information within the context of the entire patient situation.

Providing deliberate practice using a rule in a contextual manner (applied to the individual patient's situation) is one of the major purposes of this book. All nurses think contextually by engaging in situation-based thinking. This book helps students become situation-based thinkers.

During the first term (quarter, trimester, semester, etc.) of nursing courses, students begin to learn how the rules they are learning are applied to an individual patient considering all aspects of the patient situation. This thinking must be done before the nurse makes a decision. Students learn that simply applying a rule to all situations without considering the context of the patient leads to faulty thinking and poor decisions. Although novices are able to readily identify patient data, they are unable to identify important cues, especially as the complexity of a situation increases. The novice applies the rule regardless of the situation in large part due to an inability to differentiate what is important from what is not important (Koharchik, et al., 2015). **Another major goal of this book is for students to learn how to determine what information in a patient situation should be considered and how to use that information to make situation-based decisions.** Using situation-based thinking is fundamental to safe patient care and is the important cognitive process of "Analyzing Cues" that is measured on the Next Generation NCLEX.

Once you learn the "grey" lesson by applying rules within a variety of patient contexts and in a variety of healthcare environments, you are ready to be guided into and through the Advanced Beginner Stage of the Novice to Expert theory. In this stage you encounter additional experiences using rules in real and/or simulated situations to move from simple rules to guide behavior to applying principles to guide actions. You practice applying rules and learning about aspects of a situation that are relevant, and aspects of a situation that are not relevant, based on a specific patient situation. As you work through these types of experiences, you begin to use clinical judgment based on the specifics of a situation; that is, decisions made and actions taken become situation-driven rather than rule-driven.

At this point it is helpful to use learning activities that provide opportunities to apply rules to individual patient situations. This book provides those learning activities. You will compare and contrast patients with similar conditions to discover individual patient nuances (patient-specific differences) that contribute to situation-based thinking rather than rule-based thinking. In so doing, you begin to learn differences among patients who appear similar but are quite different based on the specifics of the patient context.

This way of thinking is at the heart of patient-centered care: determining nursing actions based on the collected patient information within the context of the entire patient situation.

Using situation-based thinking is fundamental to safe patient care and is the important cognitive process of "Analyzing Cues" that is measured on the Next Generation NCLEX.

The last three stages of the Novice to Expert theory are completed after graduating from nursing school and entering the nursing profession. These stages are competent, proficient, and expert. It takes approximately five years working in a profession to achieve the expert level.

COMPONENT #2

STEPS IN CLINICAL JUDGMENT

As shown in Figure 2.1, a second component of clinical judgment delineates the steps in thinking. The Caputi Clinical Judgment Framework builds on two approaches from the nursing education literature. The first approach is the Tanner Clinical Judgment Model (2006) and the second is the NCSBN Clinical Judgment Measurement Model (CJMM) (NCSBN, 2019).

The Tanner Clinical Judgment Model

TANNER CLINICAL JUDGMENT MODEL

Noticing

Interpreting

Responding

Reflecting

The Tanner Clinical Judgment Model (2006) breaks down thinking into four steps:

1. Noticing
2. Interpreting
3. Responding
4. Reflecting

These four steps represent the general, global thinking processes used by nurses. Although the steps are described as separate, distinct steps, these steps do not always flow in a linear fashion. That is, the nurse may notice something about a patient situation that represents a real or potential problem then interpret that situation as an issue. However, during the interpreting stage, the nurse may return to the noticing step to collect additional information.

The Tanner Clinical Judgment Model was very helpful in establishing a framework of general thinking used by the nurse. This model has been used to teach thinking for the last 15 years. The model is research- and evidence-based. It is a good model to use for the general steps in thinking.

The weakness of the Tanner Clinical Judgment Model is that it is not specific. What thinking does a nurse do in the Noticing step, in the Interpreting step, etc.? Students need more specific information about how to think than offered in the Tanner model. These general steps are used as part of the researched-based support for the Caputi Clinical Judgment Framework. Table 2.1 demonstrates the direct connection between Tanner's Clinical Judgment Model and the steps of the Caputi Clinical Judgment Framework. The Caputi Clinical Judgment Framework is discussed in detail later in this chapter.

TABLE 2.1

Comparing the Caputi Clinical Judgment Framework to the Tanner Clinical Judgment Model

Major Steps in the Caputi Clinical Judgment Framework	Tanner's Clinical Judgment Model
Getting the Information	Noticing
Making Meaning of the Information	Interpreting
Determining Actions to Take	No Step in the Tanner Model
Taking Action	Responding
Evaluating Outcomes and Your Thinking	Reflecting

The NCSBN's Clinical Judgment Measurement Model (CJMM)

The NGN (the new NCLEX exam) focuses on clinical judgment. The NCSBN (2019) developed their CJMM to **measure** the NCLEX candidate's ability to engage in clinical judgment. The specific cognitive processes measured with the CJMM are supported by the NCSBN's research that revealed how nurses think in practice. As discussed in Chapter 1, the six cognitive processes measured are:

1. **Recognize Cues**: "Identifying relevant and important information from different sources" (p. 4)
2. **Analyze Cues**: "Organizing and linking the recognized cues to the client's clinical presentation" (p. 4)
3. **Prioritize Hypotheses**: "Evaluating and ranking hypotheses according to priority (urgency, likelihood, risk, difficulty, time, etc.)" (p. 5)
4. **Generate Solutions**: "Identifying expected outcomes and using hypotheses to define a set of interventions for the expected outcomes" (p. 5)
5. **Take Actions**: "Implementing the solution(s) that address the highest priorities" (p. 6)
6. **Evaluate Outcomes**: "Comparing observed outcomes against expected outcomes" (p. 6)

NCSBN's
CLINICAL JUDGMENT
MEASUREMENT MODEL
(CJMM)

Recognize Cues

Analyze Cues

Prioritize Hypotheses

Generate Solutions

Take Actions

Evaluate Outcomes

These cognitive processes represent the thinking nurses use to determine patient care needs or solve problems in the healthcare environment. Although these cognitive processes are listed in an order from one to six, they are not meant to be used in one direction. That is, as the nurse works through the thinking, the nurse may return to an earlier step if needed prior to completing the remaining steps. Table 2.2 demonstrates the connection between these six cognitive processes and the Caputi Clinical Judgment Framework.

TABLE 2.2

Comparing the Caputi Clinical Judgment Framework to the NCSBN's Clinical Judgment Measurement Model

Steps in the Caputi Clinical Judgment Framework	Steps in the NCSBN's Clinical Judgment Measurement Model
Getting the Information	Recognize Cues
Making Meaning of the Information	Analyze Cues
Determining Actions to Take	Prioritize Hypotheses Generate Solutions
Taking Action	Take Actions
Evaluating Outcomes and Your Thinking	Evaluate Outcomes

As with Tanner's (2009) Clinical Judgment Model, the NCSBN's (2019) CJMM presents broad categories of thinking. The specific kind of thinking that is required in each step is not addressed. It is important to remember the NCSBN's model is a **measurement model**, it is not a model for **teaching or learning** thinking. Teaching the detailed thinking that occurs in each step of the measurement model is a major responsibility of nursing education. Each nursing program must determine how to engage students in learning clinical judgment. Teaching students to think should be a requirement of all nursing programs. As a nursing education textbook, this book teaches that detailed thinking—the missing piece of clinical judgment.

Without drilling down to the detailed thinking used in each step of either of these approaches (Tanner's model or the CJMM), the student will not learn to think in a way that is needed for today's healthcare environment. This is the overall goal of the Caputi Clinical Judgment Framework—to teach students to think like a nurse.

The Caputi Clinical Judgment Framework

The Tanner Clinical Judgment Model and the NCSBN's CJMM form the evidence to support the steps of thinking in the 2022 version of the Caputi Clinical Judgment Framework. The Caputi Method uses five overall steps to learn clinical judgment:

1. Getting the Information
2. Making Meaning of the Information
3. Determining Actions to Take
4. Taking Action
5. Evaluating Outcomes and Your Thinking

CAPUTI CLINICAL JUDGMENT FRAMEWORK

Getting the Information

Making Meaning of the Information

Determining Actions to Take

Taking Action

Evaluating Outcomes and Your Thinking

Table 2.3 demonstrates the alignment of the three general approaches to clinical judgment discussed in this chapter.

TABLE 2.3

Alignment among the NCSBN's Clinical Judgment Model, the Tanner Clinical Judgment Model, and the Caputi Clinical Judgment Framework

Steps in the NCSBN's Clinical Judgment Measurement Model	Steps in Tanner's Clinical Judgment Model	Steps in the Caputi Clinical Judgment Framework
Recognize Cues	Noticing	Getting the Information
Analyze Cues	Interpreting	Making Meaning of the Information
Prioritize Hypotheses	Interpreting	Determining Actions to Take
Generate Solutions	No Step	Determining Actions to Take
Take Actions	Responding	Taking Action
Evaluate Outcomes	Reflecting	Evaluating Outcomes and Your Thinking

Step 1: Getting the Information

The "Getting the Information" step involves collecting data about the patient or a healthcare situation. The nurse uses assessment techniques such as observation and auscultation to collect data. Information is collected from all sources such as the patient, the medical history in the patient's medical record, trends in vital signs, etc. This aligns with the NCSBN's "Recognize Cues" step.

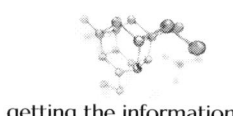

getting the information ~

collecting data about the patient or a healthcare situation

Additionally, an important skill during this step is thoughtful questioning used to explore all aspects of the situation. During the "Getting the Information" step the nurse determines information to collect to support decisions such as "all is well and going as expected," or "something is different that indicates all may not be quite right." For example, the nurse assesses the patient and collects new information that was not included in the report received from the nurse on the previous shift. Or, perhaps the nurse has learned the typical presentation of a patient with a particular medical diagnosis. However, when assessing the patient, the data demonstrate a variation from what was expected based on the nurse's report or the learned information.

There are a number of factors that affect what information the nurse collects. Three factors are:

1. the level of the nurse's knowledge
2. the nurse's prior experiences
3. personal characteristics of the nurse

The nurse's level of knowledge and prior experiences affect the information the nurse collects (NCSBN, 2019). A beginning nursing student may not collect all the necessary patient information because of unfamiliarity with many aspects of nursing. As the student learns more with each passing week, the student is better able to determine what information to collect.

Personal characteristics of the nurse also influence what information is collected (NCSBN, 2019; Nielsen & Lasater, 2021). An example of personal characteristics is preconceived ideas and attitudes. The student may enter a nursing program with many preconceived ideas and attitudes about a number of issues that can affect patient care. These preconceived ideas and attitudes greatly influence the nurse's ability when "Getting the Information." For example, if the student believes all elderly people are, to some degree, confused, then a patient's confusion may go unnoticed.

The nurse must have the self-confidence to be comfortable asking for help when unsure about what information to collect. Not noticing a problem or issue because the nurse chooses not to acknowledge they need help with the situation is an unacceptable behavior. Something about the patient's situation just doesn't seem right, but the nurse may be unable to identify or define the nature of the problem. The nurse must be comfortable asking for help and never leave a potential patient issue not identified.

An environmental factor that influences "Getting the Information" is time pressure. If the nurse is pressed for time and cannot devote the necessary time for a complete collection of patient data, information may go unnoticed. Nurses are often very busy. Learning ways to prioritize all aspects of nursing care, including "Getting the Information," can help ensure important information is not missed. Prioritizing is an important aspect of clinical judgment discussed later in this book.

The above are examples of individual and environmental factors that influence the nurse's ability to engage in the first step of the Caputi Clinical Judgment Framework, "Getting the Information." As would be expected, the more a student learns about nursing and the more nursing experiences encountered, the more astute the student will become at determining what information to collect during the "Getting the Information" step.

Step 2: Making Meaning of the Information

Once the "Getting the Information" step is complete and the data are collected, the nurse must make sense of all that information in the second step, "Making Meaning of the Information." The nurse analyzes the data to determine just what the data mean. An overall term for all the thinking of this step is **data analysis**. Nurses analyze the data to make sense of the data to determine issues, problems, or concerns. This is the NCSBN's CJMM "Analyze Cues" step in which the information is organized and linked to the patient's individual situation or context.

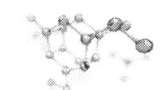

making meaning of the information ~

analyzing the data to make sense of it and to determine any issues, problems, or concerns

This is a unique step in the clinical judgment process; that is, the meaning the nurse derives from the information is dependent on a variety of factors that influence what the nurse notices. Some of the same factors that affect "Getting the Information," also affect "Making Meaning of the Information." The way the information is interpreted can differ depending on the individual nurse's background, the healthcare environment, and the patient's health situation.

The specific healthcare environment in which the patient is being cared for can affect the meaning of information collected (NCSBN, 2019; Nielsen & Lasater, 2021). For example, a laboratory value may be acceptable for a patient with a chronic illness in a long-term care environment, but the same laboratory value may not be acceptable for an acutely ill patient with no pre-existing illnesses admitted to the acute care hospital.

Because of these variables, the meaning the nurse derives from the information can vary among patients. It is most important for the information to be interpreted correctly so the planned actions will be what is needed for the specific patient situation (Nielsen & Lasater, 2021).

"Making Meaning of the Information" is a very important step because the meaning derived from the information collected determines the actions the nurse will or will not take for the patient or to solve a healthcare environment problem or situation. It is important to identify the salient (important) factors used to define the problem or situation. At this point you recall the rules, or general guidelines, such as normal ranges, steps in a nursing procedure, typical patient presentation for a specific disease process, and a multitude of other information you learned in your nursing courses. You then apply that information to interpret the information collected but within the individual patient situation. The rules or guidelines will not be strictly or absolutely applied; rather, the salient (important) aspects specific to the situation determine how that rule or guideline will be applied. Again, the more practice you have applying these rules and guidelines when "Making Meaning of the Information," the better you will become in knowing how much ambiguity (wiggle room) you have when you apply the rule or guideline.

Step 3: Determining Actions to Take

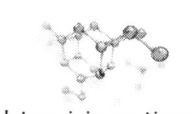

determining actions to take ~

identifying the end goal(s) often in collaboration with the patient and/or other members of the healthcare team

This step of the Caputi Clinical Judgment Framework aligns with two steps in the NCSBN's CJMM: Prioritize Hypotheses and Generate Solutions. The analysis of data in the "Making Meaning of the Information" step identifies patient care needs or problems in the healthcare environment. With the issues identified in the "Making Meaning of the Information" step, the nurse must now determine what actions to take and which actions take priority. The nurse considers what patient concerns are the most urgent, most likely to cause complications if not addressed, or at highest risk for developing into bigger concerns. These are examples of ways nurses rank patient care needs to determine which are the highest priority.

The thoughtful questioning used during the "Getting the Information" step is helpful at this point because the nurse now uses that information to explore possibilities and alternatives for care based on the individual patient context. This information is also used to prioritize patient care. The actions that are taken and how the actions are prioritized, are only as good as the information collected ("Getting the Information" step) and the meaning derived from that data ("Making Meaning of the Information" step).

When "Determining Actions to Take" the nurse must identify the end goal(s) often in collaboration with the patient and/or other members of the healthcare team. What are the expected outcomes of care? Nurses include the patient's input when establishing goals for care. What are the expected benefits from the resolution of a problem identified on the healthcare unit? Knowing the end goal(s) is critical to determining what actions to take to reach those goals.

Once the expected outcomes are determined, the nurse determines actions to take. This is the NCSBN's CJMM "Generate Solutions" step. When considering patient care concerns, the nurse draws on knowledge of identified issues and how to resolve them. For example, if the nurse determines the patient has an issue related to potential for falls, the nurse draws on knowledge of fall prevention then applies that knowledge to the individual patient situation. The patient may need assistance ambulating, or, the patient may need to learn how to use an assistive device such as a walker.

As with all steps of the clinical judgment process, the nursing actions that are planned are dependent on the patient's situation. In other words, the individual patient information used when "Making Meaning of the Information" is important for "Determining Actions to Take" that are **specific for the individual patient**. For example, you are caring for a patient who had surgery yesterday. To prevent potential complications from inactivity, you select interventions to engage the patient in various types of movement, such as changing positions in bed and ambulating. Determining how to implement the planned interventions takes place in Step 4: "Taking Action."

Step 4: Taking Action

In the "Taking Action" step the nurse carries out the nursing interventions planned during the "Determining Actions to Take" step. Those actions that were designated as the highest priority are implemented first. Actions are not just nursing interventions or psychomotor skills, but can also be delegating nursing actions for others to implement; communicating with healthcare team members; teaching patients and others; and documenting various aspects of care. How the actions are implemented are, once again, dependent on the individual patient's situation or the unique care environment.

"Taking Action" means implementing patient care in a safe manner that ensures goals are met. To determine how to take action, students recall information learned in their various nursing courses, in classroom discussions, and from prior clinical experiences. It is important for students to understand that what is learned from these sources is just one way of doing. The specifics about how any actions are implemented in the "Taking Action" step is dependent on the individual patient situation. Once again, this requires using situation-based thinking to provide for safe, effective, **individualized** patient care.

For example, based on your thinking in the first three steps, your post-operative patients must ambulate to prevent potential complications from bedrest. However, you must determine how to implement this planned intervention. How far and for how long you will ambulate each patient is affected by the factors related to the patient situation as identified in the "Making Meaning

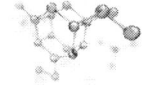

taking action ~

carrying out planned nursing interventions and implementing patient care in a safe manner that ensures goals are met

of the Information" step. "Taking Action" may involve imposing limitations related to ambulation based on the specific patient's condition. You may determine that one patient may only be able to ambulate a few feet, while another patient can ambulate much further. Making this determination is critical for safe care.

Step 5: Evaluating Outcomes and Your Thinking

As mentioned previously in the "Determining Actions to Take" step, the nurse identifies outcomes expected from the nursing care provided as determined by using clinical judgment. "Evaluating Outcomes and Your Thinking" is the last step of the clinical judgment process.

The "Evaluating Outcomes and Your Thinking" step has two parts. The first part is "Evaluating Outcomes." To "Evaluate Outcomes," the nurse:

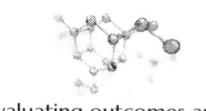

evaluating outcomes and your thinking ~

part 1:

collecting data

comparing data to determine patient's condition

planning further care

part 2:

reflecting on the process of clinical judgment/thinking to determine accuracies or areas needing improvement

1. Collects data (evaluation data) related to the effects of the nursing actions implemented for the patient. When collecting data, the nurse incorporates feedback from the patient to determine satisfaction with a specific nursing action and overall satisfaction with care delivered.

2. Compares the data collected prior to the nursing action with the data collected after implementing the nursing action. Based on this comparison, the nurse determines if the patient's condition is improving, declining, or remaining unchanged.

3. Plans further care depending on the results of #2. The nurse also considers the possibility that other nursing actions would have been more effective.

The information derived from this step drives revisions to the patient plan of care. For this reason, the nurse must ensure the accuracy of the data collected when evaluating outcomes, just as accuracy of data was ensured in the "Getting the Information" step.

The second part of the "Evaluating Outcomes and Your Thinking" step is "Evaluating Your Thinking." In this step you reflect on the thinking used throughout the entire clinical judgment process to determine if your thinking was accurate or if there are areas of thinking that need improvement. This step involves learning from your experiences by reflecting on those experiences. To improve thinking the nurse reflects on the thinking that was used throughout the clinical judgment process. Reflective thinking is tantamount to learning and growing as a nurse. Reviewing your thinking and its effectiveness encourages deeper understanding of your ability to think, supports self-evaluation, and, with honest reflection, fosters growth in your ability to use clinical judgment. There are two types of reflection that occur in this step as described by Tanner (2006).

Reflection-IN-Action

Reflection-in-action occurs while providing care for the patient or addressing the healthcare environment issue. In the case of patient care, as the nurse implements the nursing actions, the nurse continues to collect cues from the patient that indicate if the actions are, or are not, effective; or, if the actions need to be modified for this particular patient. Reflection-in-action is happening in **real time, while the nurse is providing care**. Because of the ambiguous and sometimes quickly changing patient conditions or unexpected happenings, the nurse must always consider how the patient is responding to the planned intervention while carrying out that intervention. For example, the nurse implements the plan to ambulate the patient to the nurse's station and back. However, halfway to the nurse's station, the patient becomes dizzy. The nurse will immediately revise the plan.

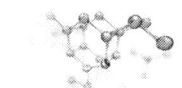

reflection-IN-action ~

occurs while providing care for the patient or addressing the healthcare environment issue

Reflection-ON-Action

As the name implies, reflection-on-action occurs upon completion of the action. This step is critical to improving clinical judgment. During this step the nurse mentally reviews what just happened to determine what went right and what went wrong. What is learned from the experience is used to improve the nurse's thinking abilities and nursing knowledge base. This is the actual learning from experience step. One does not learn by merely having an experience; one learns by reflecting on that experience. Nursing students must take time to stop and reflect on their thinking to improve their use of clinical judgment. As you engage in reflective practice to improve your clinical judgment abilities throughout your nursing program and throughout your nursing career, you will continue on your path toward the Expert Stage of Dr. Benner's Novice to Expert theory.

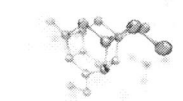

reflection-ON-action ~

occurs upon completion of the action, which is critical to improving clinical judgment

Learning Activity

Consider the five steps of the Caputi Clinical Judgment Framework. This type of thinking is not exclusive to nursing. You have likely worked through these same steps in your everyday life to solve problems. Table 2.4 presents an example of using this approach in everyday life.

TABLE 2.4

Using the Caputi Clinical Judgment Framework to Make Decisions in Everyday Life ~ Example I

BRIEF EXPLANATION OF PROBLEM:
A friend stops by and is very upset. She is crying because she needs a dress for an unexpected occasion, but can't afford to buy one.

Step in the Caputi Clinical Judgment Framework	Explanation of this Step in Solving the Problem
Getting the Information	What you know about this person: She works hard; saves money; helps her family as much as she can.
Making Meaning of the Information	You know this person and how she may react because of past experiences, so you use this information as you plan your response.
Determining Actions to Take	You decide to offer to buy the dress for her and let her decide how she will pay you back.
Taking Action	You carry out the planned actions that are individualized for this friend based on what you know of the situation and know of her. You lend her the money to buy the dress.
Evaluating Outcomes and Your Thinking	Your friend was unable to pay you back as planned, so you changed your approach slightly and offered her an additional month to pay the loan. You review in your mind how the exchange occurred and determine it went well. However, you realize that when "Determining Actions to Take" in the future you may need other alternatives for repayment of any loans to this friend.

Table 2.5 presents a similar, but somewhat different, situation. That is, the characteristics of the friend (context or situation) are a little different.

TABLE 2.5

Using the Caputi Clinical Judgment Framework to Make Decisions in Everyday Life ~ Example 2

BRIEF EXPLANATION OF PROBLEM:
A friend stops by and is very upset. She also needs a dress for the same unexpected occasion as the first friend, but also can't afford to buy one. She knows you are very supportive of your friends and asks if you can lend her the money.

Step in the Caputi Clinical Judgment Framework	Explanation of this Step in Solving the Problem
Getting the Information	What you know about this person: She spends money every day and doesn't save. She is known to borrow from others and often does not repay them or only repays them if the lender makes frequent requests for payment.
Making Meaning of the Information	You know this friend has a recurring problem that is self-imposed, so providing money each time she asks is not a good solution. Teaching the friend how to help herself would be more helpful for this occasion and for the future.
Determining Actions to Take	You decide the best way to help this friend is to take actions that will help her learn so she will be more responsible in the future. You decide to loan her a dress to wear but not to loan her money to buy something new.
Taking Action	You offer to lend her a dress to wear for the event. You explain to her that you are unable to lend her money at this time. You explore whether she would like you to teach her about how to budget her money so she can be prepared for unexpected occasions in the future.
Evaluating Outcomes and Your Thinking	Although the friend is upset about the decision not to lend her money, she has a recurring problem that is self-imposed. Providing money each time she asks is not a good solution. Teaching the friend how to help herself is more helpful. Because she declined the offer to help her budget her money, plan to engage her in future conversations about budgeting money when she does not have an immediate need. The friend decides to wear a dress she had previously purchased, but had never worn, eliminating the need to buy a new one. The thinking process used was effective in helping the friend resolve her own problem without relying on others and perhaps causing an issue that could interfere with the continued friendship.

Using Table 2.6, provide an example how you have used the steps of the Caputi Clinical Judgment Framework (CCJF) to solve a problem in your life. This does not have to be a big problem, but can be one of the many situations you face and must resolve on a daily basis.

Think through your experience and determine which actions align with each of the steps in the framework.

TABLE 2.6

Your Own Explanation of Using the 5 Steps of Clinical Judgment in Everyday Life

BRIEF EXPLANATION OF PROBLEM:

Step in the CCJF	Explanation of this Step in Solving the Problem
Getting the Information	
Making Meaning of the Information	
Determining Actions to Take	
Taking Action	
Evaluating Outcomes and Your Thinking	

Developing this ability to reflect on your thinking and use the results of your reflective thinking to improve your thinking continues throughout your nursing career. Because the healthcare environment is ever-changing and patients are different in so many ways, learning to think never ceases. Therefore, you must develop this process and become a reflective practitioner. Remember, do not just reflect on negative results. Nurses often focus on negative outcomes and work to determine how to improve (Nielsen & Lasater, 2021). Although reflecting on negative outcomes is a critical piece of reflection, so is reflection on your positive results. It is important to contemplate how what you did worked well in the situation and how it might be used or perhaps revised for use in the future. Focusing on your positive achievements as well as areas that need improvement helps you to become resilient as discussed in Chapter 1.

Although reflecting on negative outcomes is a critical piece of reflection, so is reflection on your positive results.

COMPONENT #3

CLINICAL JUDGMENT COMPETENCIES

The third component of the Caputi Clinical Judgment Framework is a listing of the specific thinking skills and strategies used in each step of the clinical judgment framework. These thinking skills and strategies are known as **clinical judgment competencies. Clinical judgment competencies are the heart of the Caputi Clinical Judgment Framework. Learning the clinical judgment competencies has been the piece missing when students are taught thinking in nursing. These competencies are the details of clinical judgment. Without learning the clinical judgment competencies, you cannot learn clinical judgment. You must learn all the clinical judgment competencies before you can use clinical judgment.**

What is a competency? A competency is a behavior. Many behaviors make up a bigger entity. In the case of the Caputi Clinical Judgment Framework, there are a number of competencies for each step. These competencies are the building blocks of the clinical judgment framework—the bigger entity. You can think of the five steps as the frame and the many clinical judgment competencies as the building blocks that lie within the frame to make it one cohesive clinical judgment process. Table 2.7 lists the steps of the Caputi Clinical Judgment Framework and the clinical judgment competencies that make up each step. These 23 clinical judgment competencies are the components of the bigger entity of clinical judgment. Clinical judgment without these clinical judgment competencies is just an empty shell. The clinical judgment competencies are the heart and soul of the clinical judgment process.

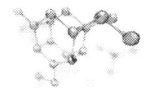

competencies ~ the specific thinking skills and strategies used in each step of the clinical judgment framework

TABLE 2.7

The Caputi Clinical Judgment Framework with Competencies

Major Steps in the Caputi Clinical Judgment Framework	The Caputi Clinical Judgment Competencies
1. Getting the Information	• Determining important information to collect • Scanning the environment • Identifying signs and symptoms • Assessing systematically and comprehensively • Ensuring accurate information
2. Making Meaning of the Information	• Clustering related information • Identifying assumptions • Recognizing inconsistencies • Distinguishing relevant from irrelevant information • Judging how much ambiguity is acceptable • Comparing and contrasting • Predicting potential complications • Collaborating with healthcare team members • Determining patient care needs/healthcare environment issues
3. Determining Actions to Take	• Selecting interventions • Managing potential complications • Setting priorities
4. Taking Action	• Determining how to implement the planned interventions • Delegating • Communicating • Teaching others
5. Evaluating Outcomes and Your Thinking	• Evaluating data • Evaluating and correcting thinking

Student behaviors that demonstrate the use of each clinical judgment competency can be measured and evaluated to determine the student's use of clinical judgment. Based on how a student performs using each of the clinical judgment competencies, nursing faculty can provide detailed, specific feedback the student can use to become a better thinker. Faculty can reinforce strong performance of the use of a particular clinical judgment competency. Faculty can also provide feedback on a competency that needs improvement and can help guide the student to better performance.

Breaking down the larger process of clinical judgment into the clinical judgment competencies is a good way to learn clinical judgment. As the student progresses through the nursing program, the student learns to use these clinical judgment competencies, not as separate ways to think, but as pieces of the larger process of clinical judgment. But to first learn the process, these individual competencies must be learned, practiced, applied to patient care, and reviewed in all learning environments.

As discussed in Chapter 1, the process of learning clinical judgment is similar to learning a nursing skill. When you learn to perform a nursing skill you are taught a step-by-step process. You learn to perform each step in the procedure. Once you learn and practice the procedure many times, you will eventually perform the procedure as a complete whole rather than as individual steps. You will also be able to safely make changes in the procedure to meet individual patient needs. This is the same approach with learning clinical judgment. You first learn all the pieces and the step-by-step process. You practice clinical judgment over and over, then eventually use clinical judgment as a whole process rather than using each individual competency, AND you will do so as needed for the individual patient situation. As previously mentioned, considering the individual patient situation is what many faculty mean when they ask the student to "look at the bigger picture." This is precisely why it is best to learn clinical judgment at the beginning of your nursing studies. You will have time to practice using clinical judgment throughout the nursing program applied to many patient situations. You will learn to think on your own while considering the "bigger picture." That is the end goal—becoming a self-directed thinker to provide individualized, safe, patient-centered care, as discussed in Chapter 1.

Think back to the earlier discussion on the advantage of having a common language to use to explain your thinking. Breaking down clinical judgment into its parts means learning **specific** clinical judgment competencies. Learning these clinical judgment competencies (thinking skills and strategies) and applying them to nursing is fundamental because once learned, the same thinking process is applied to **all** patient care environments. Nurses use the same thinking (clinical judgment) no matter the type of patient care unit. That is, the same framework for thinking is used in maternal/child, long-term care, medical-surgical, critical care, home care, and on any other type of unit where the nurse may work. These clinical judgment competencies provide the language you need to track your thinking then explain your thinking in all nursing situations.

THE END GOAL ~
to become a
self-directed thinker
to provide
individualized, safe,
patient-centered care.

Let's go back to what was mentioned in Chapter 1: Answering a question correctly does not mean you used clinical judgment; and if you did, you may not be able to explain the thinking you used. You may have discovered the answer to a question using thinking, but may not be able to explain how you arrived at the answer because you have not specifically learned the clinical judgment competencies you used to address the question. You may not have the knowledge base and the language related to clinical judgment competencies that is needed to answer the question and be able to **explain** your thinking. This book provides the language of clinical judgment through use of the clinical judgment competencies. This book also provides you practice using the clinical judgment competencies so you will become skilled at using the clinical judgment competencies and be able to use them to explain your thinking. To become skilled using the clinical judgment competencies requires using this framework throughout your entire nursing program.

Table 2.7 lists a total of 23 clinical judgment competencies nurses use. It is critical for you to learn these competencies that are used to think like a nurse so you are able to explain your thinking. This critical piece is often missing.

This book provides specific guidance for applying clinical judgment competencies in clinical situations. In both the critical thinking and nursing education literature, there are many thinking skills identified that form the basis for the clinical judgment competencies (Caputi, 2010a; 2010b; Lasater, 2011; Paul & Elder, 2020). The chapters in Section I of this book present the clinical judgment competencies and provide activities you can use to apply them to nursing. These activities guide your thinking. These activities provide you with the practice needed to become a skilled thinker.

You must not only learn what these clinical judgment competencies are but must actually use them in clinical situations. Through this process you learn what is meant by "nursing is not black or white, but grey." This book offers many activities to apply these thinking skills in the classroom, the simulation laboratory, and the clinical setting. These activities engage you in using the clinical judgment competencies in a way that enables your faculty to use concrete language to provide the necessary feedback on your use of the clinical judgment competencies as you grow in your ability to think.

Putting the Three Components Together

None of the three individual components alone can result in learning how to think like a nurse. They all work together to develop your thinking using clinical judgment across time. You will use the five steps of Caputi Clinical Judgment Framework to organize your thinking then use clinical judgment competencies when working through each step.

As you become skilled using the clinical judgment competencies, you will move through Benner's Novice Stage entering the Advanced Beginner Stage. Engaging in deliberate practice using the clinical judgment activities in the book requires you to apply clinical judgment to individual patient care and to deal with other nursing situations. This application of what you are learning about clinical judgment will help you transition from Novice to Advanced Beginner. You move from rule-based thinking (Novice Stage) to situation-based thinking (Advanced Beginner Stage).

The Nursing Process and the Caputi Clinical Judgment Framework

In all pre-licensure nursing programs students learn the nursing process. The nursing process is another step-by-step process to guide nursing decisions. The five steps of the nursing process are:

1. Assessing
2. Diagnosing
3. Planning
4. Implementing
5. Evaluating

FIVE STEPS OF
THE NURSING PROCESS

Assessing

Diagnosing

Planning

Implementing

Evaluating

The nursing process is still in use today and will be used in the foreseeable future. Some sources may suggest that the NCSBN's CJMM replaces the nursing process. This is absolutely not the case. Suggesting that the CJMM replaces the nursing process represents a misunderstanding of what the CJMM is all about.

Consider the five steps listed above. As with the six cognitive processes of the NCSBN's CJMM, these five steps represent general, overall thinking the nurse uses. Because these are general steps, they do not represent the detailed thinking the nurse uses. This is where the clinical judgment competencies once again are needed. Think of the Caputi Clinical Judgment Framework as **the thinking behind** the five general steps of the nursing process.

Table 2.8 aligns the NCSBN's CJMM cognitive processes, the steps of the Caputi Clinical Judgment Framework, and the steps of the Nursing Process.

TABLE 2.8

Alignment of the NCSBN Clinical Judgment Measurement Model, the Caputi Clinical Judgment Framework, and the Steps of the Nursing Process

The Cognitive Processes of the NCSBN Clinical Judgment Measurement Model	Major Steps in the Caputi Clinical Judgment Framework	Steps of the Nursing Process
1. Recognize Cues	Getting the Information	Assessing
2. Analyze Cues	Making Meaning of the Information	Diagnosing
3. Prioritize Hypotheses	Determining Actions to Take	Planning
4. Generate Solutions	Determining Actions to Take	Planning
5. Take Actions	Taking Action	Implementing
6. Evaluate Outcomes	Evaluating Outcomes and Your Thinking	Evaluating

NOTE OF CLARIFICATION

The diagnosing step in the nursing process involves the nurse interpreting the data collected, making meaning of the data, then determining individual patient care needs (issues, problems, concerns). The verbiage used to make a nursing diagnosis varies. For example, some nursing schools use the North American Nursing Diagnosis Association (NANDA) verbiage. However, when a nurse makes a nursing diagnosis, that act does not automatically mean NANDA verbiage is used. Some nursing programs teach students to state the nursing diagnosis related to patient issues, concerns, and problems in the form of a concept, such as an issue with nutrition or perfusion. Healthcare organizations are trending toward not using NANDA, but instead stating nursing diagnoses in terms of problems or issues identified, which is especially helpful when collaborative patient care notes are written. Students must consult with their nursing programs to determine how to state the nursing diagnosis—in NANDA terms or in terms of issues identified. The NCLEX has never tested NANDA verbiage. The NCSBN has indicated that remains true for the Next Generation NCLEX. Therefore, learning NANDA verbiage is not necessary to pass the NCLEX.

It is important that all nursing students understand the nursing process is a cornerstone of nursing practice. It is what is used every day by nurses. The cognitive processes of the NCSBN's CJMM and the steps of the Caputi Clinical Judgment Framework as well as all the clinical judgment competencies represent the thinking used to implement the nursing process. As you become a self-directed thinker and eventually move into the Expert level of practice, the language of clinical judgment will fade; however, the thinking will be automatic and ever present. Yet the language of the steps of the nursing process will continue to guide nursing practice. **Clinical judgment does not replace the nursing process; it is the thinking that supports the nurse's use of the nursing process.**

Clinical judgment does not replace the nursing process; it is the thinking that supports the nurse's use of the nursing process.

ANOTHER NOTE OF CLARIFICATION

The nursing process is used to identify, plan, and evaluate nursing care related to individual patient needs. As noted, the Caputi Clinical Judgment Framework is the thinking behind that process. However, the Caputi Clinical Judgment Framework is a thinking framework that is also used to solve problems and address issues on the healthcare unit, not just those related to a patient. The nursing process is used for patient-related situations; the Caputi Clinical Judgment Framework is used for patient-related situations as well as to address all other issues, problems, and concerns that may not be directly related to a patient. For example, the thinking process as presented in the Caputi Clinical Judgment Framework can be used to address conflicts between healthcare providers or issues related to managing a care unit. Therefore, the Caputi Clinical Judgment Framework is a method for thinking that can be used to address a variety of healthcare issues and is not limited to use with patient care. The Caputi Clinical Judgment Framework provides a thinking process that can be applied to all nursing situations.

Chapter 2 Summary

The Caputi Clinical Judgment Framework is fairly simple. What sets the Caputi Clinical Judgment Framework apart from other approaches that are used to teach students to think like a nurse can be summarized as follows:

1. Learn individual clinical judgment competencies.

2. Engage in deliberate, focused practice to apply each of the clinical judgment competencies in the classroom, the simulation laboratory, and clinical experiences.

3. Demonstrate progression through the thinking of a Novice and into the Advanced Beginner stage.

4. Continue this process across the curriculum.

Many resources for teaching nursing students to think present case studies then ask students to answer questions. If the student answers the questions correctly, it is assumed the student knows how to think like a nurse. As presented thus far in this book, it is obvious that is an incorrect conclusion and does not help the student learn to think like a nurse.

The end goal of implementing a deliberate method for learning clinical judgment is improved patient outcomes. As a new graduate applying for a first nursing position, you must be able to talk this talk.

During an interview for a nursing position, as you share all the psychomotor skills you performed while in the clinical setting throughout school, you should also share all the specific processes you learned for thinking including all the clinical judgment competencies you learned and applied for the purpose of:

- Enhancing patient safety
- Identifying patient care needs
- Identifying potential complications
- Decreasing the failure to rescue rate
- Improving patient outcomes
- Dealing with issues in the healthcare environment

These are the reasons why you are learning clinical judgment and why you are studying this textbook.

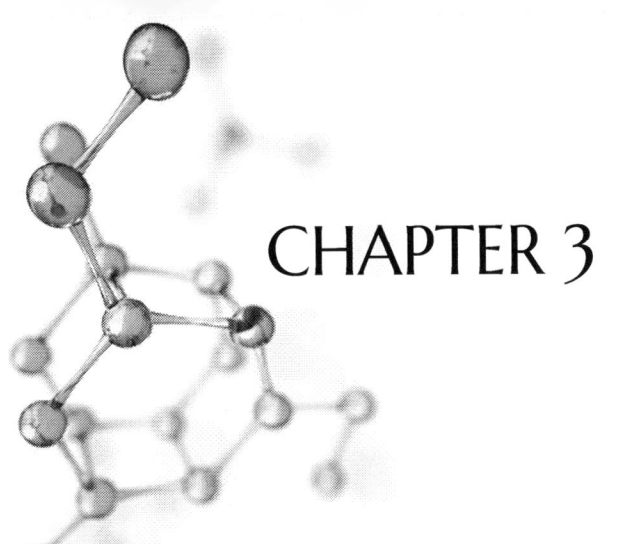

CHAPTER 3

Step 1: Getting the Information (NCLEX®~Recognize Cues)

TABLE 3.1

The Caputi Clinical Judgment Framework ~ Step 1

Major Steps in the Caputi Clinical Judgment Framework	The Caputi Clinical Judgment Competencies
STEP 1 ~ Getting the Information	• Determining important information to collect • Scanning the environment • Identifying signs and symptoms • Assessing systematically and comprehensively • Ensuring accurate information
STEP 2 ~ Making Meaning of the Information	• Clustering related information • Identifying assumptions • Recognizing inconsistencies • Distinguishing relevant from irrelevant information • Judging how much ambiguity is acceptable • Comparing and contrasting • Predicting potential complications • Collaborating with healthcare team members • Determining patient care needs/healthcare environment issues
STEP 3 ~ Determining Actions to Take	• Selecting interventions • Managing potential complications • Setting priorities
STEP 4 ~ Taking Action	• Determining how to implement the planned interventions • Delegating • Communicating • Teaching others
STEP 5 ~ Evaluating Outcomes and Your Thinking	• Evaluating data • Evaluating and correcting thinking

Think Like a Nurse: The Caputi Method for Learning Clinical Judgment

> *Nurses must be information seekers; they must dig deeper to discover all the relevant information related to a particular situation or patient care need.*

As shown in Table 3.1, this chapter presents the clinical judgment competencies under Step 1: "Getting the Information" of the Caputi Clinical Judgment Framework. This step is all about information seeking. The nurse recognizes cues that are obvious and familiar to the nurse. However, once those obvious and familiar cues are identified, the nurse must dig deeper to seek additional information related to those familiar cues. This is often an area of data collection that is difficult for newly graduated nurses unless they have had practice using the clinical judgment competencies of Step 1: "Getting the Information." Nurses must be information seekers; they must dig deeper to discover all the relevant information related to a particular situation or patient care need. All relevant information must be collected. Many of the clinical judgment competencies in Step 1 help you develop information-seeking abilities.

Table 3.2 demonstrates how the "Getting the Information" step aligns with the NCSBN's Clinical Judgment Measurement Model cognitive process of "Recognize Cues" (NCSBN, 2019) and the Assessing step of the nursing process. **Remember**, the Caputi Clinical Judgment Framework is the detailed thinking of the six cognitive processes that are tested on the Next Generation NCLEX and the thinking behind the nursing process. The Caputi Clinical Judgment Framework does not replace the nursing process; it provides the detailed thinking needed to accurately implement the nursing process.

TABLE 3.2

Alignment of the NCSBN Clinical Judgment Measurement Model, the Caputi Clinical Judgment Framework, and the Steps of the Nursing Process

The Cognitive Processes of the NCSBN Clinical Judgment Measurement Model (Next Generation NCLEX)	Major Steps in the Caputi Clinical Judgment Framework	Steps of the Nursing Process
1. Recognize Cues	Getting the Information	Assessing
2. Analyze Cues	Making Meaning of the Information	Diagnosing
3. Prioritize Hypotheses	Determining Actions to Take	Planning
4. Generate Solutions	Determining Actions to Take	Planning
5. Take Actions	Taking Action	Implementing
6. Evaluate Outcomes	Evaluating Outcomes and Your Thinking	Evaluating

The "Recognize Cues" cognitive process of the NCSBN Clinical Judgment Measurement Model (the part of NLCEX that tests clinical judgment) refers to the nurse collecting information to use to determine the care the patient needs or to approach a healthcare environment problem. But what kind of thinking does the nurse use to "Recognize Cues?" Students cannot be instructed to visit the patient and "Recognize Cues" without learning the kind of thinking required to recognize cues. That is why learning the clinical judgment competencies is so important—these competencies inform the nurse about the thinking required to recognize cues. The clinical judgment competencies (thinking skills) under Step 1: "Getting the Information" direct students in their thinking to enable them to know how to "Recognize Cues." Preparing for the NCLEX starts now. Learning the clinical judgment competencies that enable you to "Recognize Cues" is the beginning step as you prepare throughout your program to take the NCLEX.

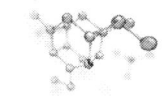

recognize cues ~

collecting information to use to determine the care the patient needs or to approach a healthcare environment problem

Table 3.3 lists the specific thinking skills (clinical judgment competencies) that are needed to be skillful at implementing the "Recognize Cues" cognitive process of the NCSBN's Clinical Judgment Measurement Model. It will be difficult to "Recognize Cues" without learning the detailed thinking that supports that type of thinking.

TABLE 3.3

Recognize Cues (Next Gen NCLEX Cognitive Process) Aligned to the Clinical Judgment Competencies of "Getting the Information"

NCSBN's Clinical Judgment Measurement Model Cognitive Process	Clinical Judgment Competencies in Caputi's "Getting the Information" Step
Recognize Cues	Determining important information to collect
	Scanning the environment
	Identifying signs and symptoms
	Assessing systematically and comprehensively
	Ensuring accurate information

Nurses typically do not use one thinking competency at a time, but use many thinking competencies to solve a problem.

It is important to understand that each clinical judgment competency of this step (and all the steps) may be used in steps other than the one in which it is presented; however, for organizational and learning purposes the thinking competencies that best align with a specific step are presented under that step. **It is critical to note that nurses typically do not use one thinking competency at a time, but use many thinking competencies to solve a problem.** Learn each of the competencies and use them in the steps as presented in this book. Applying these thinking competencies one at a time as you learn them allows careful study of the clinical judgment process. That is, clinical judgment is unpacked so you can learn how to think.

With more experience, once you master this organized method for thinking, you will use the clinical judgment competencies in this same order, or at times, you will use a specific competency as needed no matter in which step you are working. This method for learning clinical judgment is flexible.

How the Content is Presented

The information about each clinical judgment competency presented in this chapter is organized as follows:

1. Definition of the clinical judgment competency
2. Example using that clinical judgment competency in everyday life
3. Example using that clinical judgment competency in a nursing situation
4. A cognitive guidance tool (thinking activity) to use with a patient in the clinical setting to apply the clinical judgment competency in a real-world setting

Learning each competency in this manner provides information about the clinical judgment competency, presents an example of using it in your everyday life and within nursing, then gives you an opportunity to actually use that clinical judgment competency in real nursing practice. It is important to work through these activities in an actual clinical setting to reinforce and apply your learning. Immediate application of your learning is most helpful for deep learning with easier recall of that learning when needed in future situations.

But do these activities really work? Can't I just learn by reading the book? It is not enough to learn the knowledge presented in this book about thinking. Like all knowledge in nursing education, just knowing information does not always mean the nurse knows ***how to use*** the information when needed. Knowing how to use nursing knowledge within an individual patient context is the basis for safe nursing care. Just learning the knowledge is never enough; knowing how to use that knowledge when needed in a specific situation is what nurses must be able to do. This is why practice with these thinking activities is so very much needed. This is the same as learning and perfecting psychomotor skills such as administering medications or changing a dressing. You must practice, practice, practice! Applying thinking in a new discipline is not intuitive and automatic; it takes practice, practice, practice!

These practice activities are critical to learning how to think using clinical judgment. These activities can be viewed as scripts, or as organized ways to approach a situation or a problem (Panadero, et al., 2013). This process is enhanced with well-designed, thoughtful questions and inquiries about thinking as you work through the activity (Lasater, 2011). Just as you learn a nursing psychomotor skill by reviewing the steps of the procedure and applying those steps during practice, learning how to think like a nurse is enhanced with a similar approach. What you are learning in this book is a method to organize your thinking (which you already know how to do) to apply to nursing situations you encounter (which is new to you).

As the nurse you will be required to determine which clinical judgment competencies are needed to make decisions and address patient needs. At first this process is very deliberate, with careful thinking required throughout each step. However, the more practice you have with deliberate use of the clinical judgment competencies, the more automatic your thinking in nursing becomes just as thinking in your everyday life is automatic. This is why practice using these competencies is so important; frequent deliberate practice leads to automatic, self-directed thinking. That is the end goal for learning the Caputi Method for Learning Clinical Judgment—to become a **self-directed thinker**. You will direct your own thinking—rather than relying on your faculty asking you the questions you need to think about. You must learn to determine what questions to ask yourself. This goal can be accomplished by using the Caputi Clinical Judgment Framework.

Knowing how to use nursing knowledge within an individual patient context is the basis for safe nursing care.

Applying thinking in a new discipline is not intuitive and automatic; it takes PRACTICE, PRACTICE, PRACTICE.

Using the Clinical Judgment Competencies

As discussed earlier, while applying the clinical judgment competencies of the "Getting the Information" step, the nurse identifies cues or information to use to identify issues or concerns, then determines actions to take. However, what information or content is noticed or recognized depends on:

1. The nurse's knowledge base

2. Personal characteristics of the nurse such as preconceived attitudes and self-confidence

3. The context of the situation—the individual patient situation or specific healthcare setting; that is, what is meaningful in one situation may not be meaningful in another

The nurse's knowledge base might include knowledge about diagnostic tests, the physiology of body systems, pathophysiology of diseases, and concepts used in nursing practice. As you collect data during this step of clinical judgment, think about and question your knowledge base.

- What do you know?

- What do you need to know? Are there holes in your knowledge base?

- What information do you need to find out to address the problem?

- What do you need to review in a reference book to determine what information to collect and the significance of the data you are collecting?

- What sources of information will you use?

- Are there any monitors or alarms in place that provide information about the patient's condition? Do you need to learn about this equipment?

Assessing your own knowledge base and identifying sources to augment that knowledge is an important activity as you are using the clinical judgment competencies of Step 1: "Getting the Information."

As you work through the clinical judgment activities (cognitive guidance tools) in clinical situations, you will need to **apply content** you are learning in your nursing courses. If you are unsure of the content, use reliable resources to locate the information needed to work through the thinking. Some of those resources include:

1. Your own previous learning and experience in nursing
2. Previous practice using thinking in everyday life and in nursing
3. Your patient's medical record
4. Nursing textbooks
5. Online resources including reliable websites
6. Policy and procedure manuals
7. Published professional standards including your state nurse practice act providing information on scope of practice
8. Job descriptions
9. The nurse with whom you are working
10. Your teacher/preceptor
11. Evidence-based nursing resources

These are examples of sources of information. Other sources of information may be available depending on the situation.

"Getting the Information" (Recognize Cues) Clinical Judgment Competencies

This first step of clinical judgment forms the basis for the next steps of the clinical judgment process. There are five clinical judgment competencies in the "Getting the Information" step presented in this chapter:

1. Determining important information to collect
2. Scanning the environment
3. Identifying signs and symptoms
4. Assessing systematically and comprehensively
5. Ensuring accurate information

STEP 1: Getting the Information

CLINICAL JUDGMENT COMPETENCIES

DETERMINING IMPORTANT INFORMATION TO COLLECT

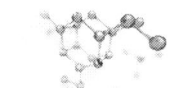

determining important information ~

collecting data that will affect the plan of the initial care of the patient as well as what information requires vigilant monitoring of the patient

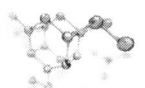

failure to rescue ~

when a patient's situation has deteriorated to the point of severe consequences or even death

Vigilant monitoring of important information contributes to the prevention of untoward events from happening.

Definition of "Determining Important Information" to Collect

The world produces an endless supply of information. The barrage of general information can be overwhelming. It is important to sort out all the information one encounters in a day by determining what information deserves attention and what information does not deserve attention. Additionally, when an issue presents itself, it is important to determine what information is important to consider related to that issue. Without doing so the person becomes overwhelmed and the issue may not be resolved.

The ability to determine important information on which to focus is an attribute of resilience as discussed in Chapter 1. As defined in Chapter 1, resilience is "the capacity to accurately perceive and respond well to stressful situations" (Sieg, 2020, para. 2). *Determining Important Information to Collect* contributes to accurately perceiving a situation. Knowing what information to collect is important, especially when faced with a stressful situation.

Nurses face myriad information to sort through for every patient. The initial processing of this information requires knowing what information is important. Additionally, patient information may change, often throughout the course of a day. Therefore, nurses must be able to determine what information to collect that is important to plan the initial care of the patient as well as what information requires vigilant monitoring of the patient. That is, the nurse must determine what information is important to collect throughout the day to identify any changes in the patient's condition. The nurse uses this information to determine if the patient's condition is improving, staying the same, or deteriorating. This is important thinking for the nurse to ensure the patient's situation is not deteriorating to the point of severe consequences and even death. This is called "failure to rescue." Vigilant monitoring of important information contributes to the prevention of untoward events from happening.

Determining Important Information to Collect is the initial clinical judgment competency of the "Getting the Information" step. Knowledge of what information to collect will be used with other clinical judgment competencies of this step such as: *Scanning the Environment, Identifying Signs and Symptoms,* and *Assessing Systematically and Comprehensively*.

Example Using "Determining Important Information to Collect" in Everyday Life

Every day one needs to determine what information to collect in many different situations. For example, you are at the Newark, New Jersey airport scheduled on a direct, nonstop flight to the Los Angeles Airport (LAX). Your plane is delayed an hour, then another hour. Finally, the airline announces the flight has been canceled. You must now *Determine Important Information to Collect* to determine what flights are available that you may attempt to book for the purpose of arriving at your destination on the same day as you originally planned. There is a lot of information to sort through to determine what data are important to help meet your goal.

You immediately start to collect important information to try to arrive in Los Angeles today as intended. You collect information about:

1. Direct flights on your scheduled airline going to Los Angeles
2. Connecting flights on your scheduled airline going to Los Angeles
3. Flights on your scheduled airline going to other Los Angeles airports such as the John Wayne airport or the Ontario airport
4. Flights going to Los Angeles or a nearby airport on another airline

You have approximately 10 flights that are a possibility for you to select to meet your goal of arriving in Los Angeles this evening. Once you have all this important information you will process this information using the clinical judgment competency of *Distinguishing Relevant from Irrelevant Information* in Step 2 of the Caputi Clinical Judgment Framework: "Making Meaning of the Information." We will return to this example in Chapter 4 to complete the thinking about this problem.

Thinking Challenge

Provide an example of how you use the clinical judgment competency of *Determining Important Information to Collect* in your everyday life.

Example Using "Determining Important Information to Collect" in Nursing

Prior to visiting a patient, the nurse considers important information to collect. The process for doing so involves reviewing the information shared by the nurse on the previous shift. Additionally, sources of information to consider include the patient's demographics (age, culture, etc.), any abnormal findings reported by the previous nurse, the patient's pathophysiology, and the patient's pertinent medical history. Prior to visiting the patient, many nurses also consider what the normal expectations for the patient might be. They ask themselves, "Based on what I've learned about this patient and what I know about this particular pathology, what do I expect to see when I walk in the room?" This provides somewhat of a baseline of thinking about what important information to consider for the individual patient. **Remember:** You may be assigned two patients with the same medical diagnosis but both patients bring their own individual backgrounds that impact their current situation. The care for each of these two patients may be very different. This is part of the **situation-based thinking** you learned about in Chapter 2.

You may be assigned two patients with the same medical diagnosis but both patients bring their own individual backgrounds that impact their current situation.

For example, the nurse is caring for a patient who is two days post abdominal surgery. The patient has a history of diabetes mellitus, hypertension, frequent urinary tract infections, and coronary artery disease. The nurse would quickly recall current knowledge about these conditions, then think about important information to collect related to each. The nurse also considers the patient's individual situation to determine what additional information to collect. This clinical forethought helps frame the nurse's thinking with a plan so important information is not overlooked.

Clinical forethought refers to looking ahead—determining what to think about as you anticipate patient needs and prevent problems before they occur. Clinical forethought contributes to resiliency because it helps you to be mindful about what you need to think about. Clinical forethought involving the thinking, predictions, and actions needed for a particular patient is intuitive or obvious to an experienced nurse; clinical forethought is not intuitive nor obvious to beginning nursing students. Practicing clinical forethought is a helpful habit as you learn clinical judgment.

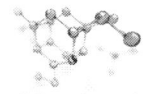

clinical forethought ~

looking ahead; determining what to think about as you anticipate patient needs and prevent problems before they occur

When visiting this patient at 0830, the patient states she is feeling a little dizzy and is somewhat confused in her thinking. Because of the clinical forethought the nurse used as well as the nurse's knowledge about the conditions the patient is experiencing, the nurse decides to check the patient's (1) blood sugar, (2) blood pressure, and (3) level of pain at the surgical site as well as any ask about any (4) chest discomfort. The nurse also (5) observes the urine in the urinary drainage bag. The nurse collected this important information in an attempt to seek information guided by the patient's medical history and pathophysiology of pre-existing conditions that may account for the new report of dizziness and slight confusion. There are other assessment data the nurse will collect for this patient relative to the patient's overall condition. Once the data are collected the nurse must determine which of the collected data are relevant. The clinical judgment competency of *Distinguishing Relevant from Irrelevant Data* as it relates to this situation is discussed in Step 2 of the Caputi Clinical Judgment Framework: "Making Meaning of the Information." We will return to this example at that time.

Cognitive Guidance Tool for the Clinical Judgment Competency of "Determining Important Information to Collect"

COGNITIVE GUIDANCE
TOOL

This tool guides your use of the clinical judgment competency of *Determining Important Information to Collect*. There are many times you will use this clinical judgment competency in a variety of situations. This tool is just one example. Fill in the information or answer the questions on a piece of paper or use an electronic device as instructed by your faculty.

The information you gather about a patient provides a total patient picture. From this information, you must determine which information is most important for the care of the patient. Many other clinical judgment competencies require application of the competency of *Determining Important Information to Collect*. To practice using this clinical judgment competency, consider the following tool as you engage in clinical forethought about what information to collect.

Basic Patient Information Important to Collect

1. **Patient information ~**
   - Age
   - Date of admission
   - Surgical procedure
   - Activity
   - Reason for admission
   - Diagnostic procedures
   - Diet
   - Vital signs
   - Trending of vital signs: *How have the vital signs changed from the previous reading; from the previous 24 hours?*

2. **Medications ~** *Complete for each medication prescribed.*
   - Drug prescribed
   - Therapeutic effects expected
   - Results the patient experienced
   - Reason why it was prescribed
   - Adverse effects to monitor

3. **Patient history** ~ *Review the patient's history. From the history, determine the most important data impacting this hospitalization and the patient's care.*

4. **Diagnostic tests** ~ *Complete for each diagnostic test ordered.*
   - Name of test
   - Why this test was ordered
   - Test results
   - Trending of the results: If the test was performed more than once, how have the results changed from the previous reading?

Answer the following questions:

Question

Was all the information you noted important to collect for this patient?

Why? Why not?

Question

Is there other information not included in the above list that you should collect?

List that information and explain why it would be important to collect that information as well.

As you progress through the nursing program you will learn more about patient care and important patient information to collect. As you continue to learn, add to this list of initial important information to collect. There is much more information you'll think about; this tool is a starting point.

As you continue your journey in learning clinical judgment, you will learn to process the above information when you engage in "Making Meaning of the Information" in Step 2.

CLINICAL JUDGMENT COMPETENCIES

SCANNING THE ENVIRONMENT

Definition of "Scanning the Environment"

Scanning the Environment means to quickly look over a location (immediate surroundings) of interest. *Scanning the Environment* involves using one's senses to perceive the elements and events in an environment. The result of *Scanning the Environment* is to understand the environmental elements and events to determine their meaning, identify any dangers or threats, and use the information to make decisions. An environmental scan provides information about unexpected occurrences. As discussed in Chapter 1, one of the reasons to learn clinical judgment is to empower you to deal with unexpected occurrences to reduce errors in the healthcare setting.

For example, when the nurse enters a patient's room, the nurse takes in the "bigger picture" of the environment, such as the equipment in place, where the patient is located, the positioning of the patient, and the presence of visitors or other health professionals at the bedside. A quick review of the area provides much information the nurse uses when working through the clinical judgment competencies of the first step of the Caputi Clinical Judgment Framework, "Getting the Information." The nurse identifies cues about additional important information to collect to add to those already identified when *Determining Important Information to Collect* prior to entering the patient's care area. The nurse has already developed a picture of what might be expected in the environment (clinical forethought), then compares that mental picture to what is actually seen.

What is expected in the environment depends on the type of healthcare setting. The environment of a long-term care setting will be quite different than an intensive care setting or the home setting. In the home setting, an additional aspect of scanning the environment includes ensuring the environment is safe for the nurse to enter and remain. A more in-depth environmental scan may involve collecting information about the general operation of a care unit. Issues that are identified may include the organization of the unit, the staffing patterns, the level of satisfaction of the nurses working on the unit, and other unit-specific information.

STEP 1:

Getting the Information

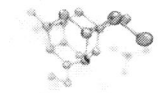

scanning the environment ~
*to quickly look over
a location
(immediate surroundings)
of interest;
use one's senses
to perceive the elements
and events in an
environment in order to
determine their meaning,
identify any dangers
or threats, and use the
information to make
decisions*

Environmental awareness is one of the environmental factors of the NCLEX Clinical Judgment Measurement Model.

There are a number of factors that can affect one's ability to engage in an environmental scan.

1. Holding false assumptions about a situation that interfere with an accurate scan
2. Poor communication when receiving information about the patient
3. Misinterpretation of information provided
4. Past experiences that cloud judgment
5. New situations that are unfamiliar This is why it is important to determine what you need to think about when you encounter a new situation. The importance of addressing your knowledge was discussed at the beginning of this chapter.
6. Pressure to get the job done
7. Other thoughts on your mind that interfere with clear thinking. This is why mindfulness as discussed in Chapter 1 is so important.

It is important to be aware of the environment. Environmental awareness is one of the environmental factors of the NCLEX Clinical Judgment Measurement Model. Another factor in that model is time pressure. As noted above, pressure to get the job done can affect the nurse's ability to conduct an environmental scan.

Example Using "Scanning the Environment" in Everyday Life

Scanning the Environment is a commonly used thinking competency in everyday life. Examples include scanning the checkout lines in a grocery store to determine which line to enter. Looking at a map on the GPS that shows traffic is a way to scan the traffic environment to determine which route to take to a destination. Another example is scanning the seating chart on a map of a theater to determine what seats are available when buying tickets to an event.

It is also important to *Scan the Environment* for safety purposes. It is common to scan the environment to locate exits when entering a crowded room. *Scanning the Environment* is also helpful when entering a party hosted by a new acquaintance in an area new to the party-goer. That person might scan the neighborhood when approaching the home, then scan the environment inside the house for any safety concerns.

Thinking Challenge

Provide an example of how you use the clinical judgment competency of *Scanning the Environment* in your everyday life.

Example Using "Scanning the Environment" in Nursing

Nurses in all care areas scan the environment. *Scanning the Environment* may involve a particular unit in a healthcare agency, the patient's room, the patient's home, or the community in which a patient lives. *Scanning the Environment* provides an overall, initial "feel" of a particular environment and the opportunity to identify any unexpected occurrences as well as determine the safety of the environment for both the nurse and the patient. Safety of the environment for the patient considers issues such as water on the floor, bedrails down, call light that is not within the patient's reach, an overfull urinary drainage bag causing urine to not properly drain, improperly positioned equipment, and small area rugs in the home environment that may slip resulting in a fall. These are just examples of the many factors that can interfere with a patient's safety that can be identified while *Scanning the Environment*.

Cognitive Guidance Tool for the Clinical Judgment Competency of "Scanning the Environment"

COGNITIVE GUIDANCE TOOL

The cognitive guidance tool for *Scanning the Environment* provides practice with this competency when entering a patient's room in the hospital or in-patient setting. There are many times you will use this clinical judgment competency in a variety of situations. This tool is just one example. Fill in the information or answer the questions on a piece of paper or use an electronic device as instructed by your faculty.

Quick Scan of the In-Patient Unit

Scanning the Environment starts outside the patient's room so as you approach the door start your environmental scan. Stand outside the patient's room making observations while performing hand hygiene and donning any required personal protective equipment (PPE).

Scanning the Environment continues upon entering the patient's room so as you walk through the door start your environmental scan. The bulk of the scan is conducted prior to starting the patient assessment, but also continues throughout your time in the room to ensure nothing is missed. Use your senses to collect the information. Ask yourself, what do you see, hear, smell, and feel?

Answer the following questions:

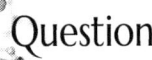
Question

What do you see?

1. Is there signage for specific infection and prevention control precautions at the doorway? Is the signage as expected or unexpected? Is the appropriate PPE stocked outside the room or in the anteroom?

2. Where is the patient? Is the patient comfortably and safely positioned?

3. Do you see any safety concerns for this patient?

4. Is the patient awake, asleep? Relaxed? Guarding? In pain or obvious distress?

5. What is the patient's facial expression? Is it relaxed? Tense? Appropriate for the situation?

6. Is there any required emergency equipment present and/or functioning (suction, emergency airways, bag-valve mask, oxygen flow meter and oxygen tubing)?

7. Is there any safety equipment in the room such as a bed alarm or floor mat sensor to indicate the patient is out of the bed?

8. What equipment is in the room? Therapeutic bed? Oxygen? IV? Other tubes? Urinary drainage? Monitors? Any specimen collection devices? Mobility aids?

9. Who besides the patient is in the room? Visitors? Other healthcare personnel? What are they doing?

10. Is the room neat, messy, food trays at the bedside?

Question

What do you hear?

1. Are there any monitors beeping? Any alarms going off?

2. Is the patient talking? Moaning? Crying? Snoring?

Question

What do you smell?

1. What smells are expected?

2. Are there any smells that are unexpected? What might those smells mean?

Question

What do you feel?

1. Is the room hot? Cold? Is the temperature what it should be for this patient?

2. Is the floor slippery? Sticky?

Conclusions:

1. Does everything seem right?

2. Does the scan indicate a problem? What might that problem be?
   Is the problem urgent? Is there an action you should take immediately?

3. Anything unexpected?

4. Did you discover anything new that you should act on during this visit or after you leave the room?

STEP 1: Getting the Information

CLINICAL JUDGMENT COMPETENCIES

IDENTIFYING SIGNS AND SYMPTOMS

Definition of "Identifying Signs and Symptoms"

Identifying Signs and Symptoms directly relates to the cognitive process of "Recognizing Cues" needed when taking the NCLEX exam. Signs and symptoms (taken together are known as clinical manifestations) represent the objective (signs) and subjective (symptoms) data collected in a situation. Signs (objective data) are data the nurse can measure or observe such as using a scale to weigh a patient. Symptoms (subjective data) are data the patient, family member, or other person tells the nurse which is not objectively measured, such as the person telling the nurse their weight. Whenever possible the nurse attempts to confirm the symptoms (subjective data reported to the nurse) with signs (objective data that can be measured to confirm the accuracy of the subjective data).

In nursing, this clinical judgment competency refers to an ability to identify the signs and symptoms of a disease (by understanding the pathophysiology), side effects of a medication, indication a treatment or intervention is working or is not working, and a host of other factors that indicate the status of a patient and/or the presence of an issue or concern for the patient. To identify signs and symptoms (clinical manifestations) the nurse must have knowledge about all the factors influencing the patient's condition and situation. Identified signs and symptoms are compared to (1) what is normal for that particular patient and (2) the patient's previous assessment. This comparison helps the nurse make decisions about the information collected as well as what further information to collect.

Identifying Signs and Symptoms is not confined to the signs and symptoms of a medical diagnosis such as pneumonia or depression. *Identifying Signs and Symptoms* also refers to areas of concerns such as the patient has a knowledge deficit requiring patient teaching, or signs of a safety hazard such as the side rails down and the bed in the high position.

The clinical judgment competency of *Identifying Signs and Symptoms* is constantly used in the clinical setting. This competency is used when performing an initial assessment of the patient, but also when working with the patient throughout the day to notice any early or subtle changes in the patient's condition. It is critical to use this clinical judgment competency for identifying

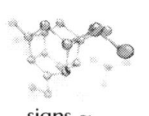

signs ~

objective data a nurse can measure or observe

symptoms ~

subjective data the patient, family member, or others tell the nurse which is not objectively measured

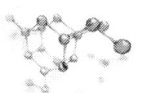

clinical manifestations ~

objective (signs) and subjective (symptoms) data collected together in a clinical situation

changes in the patient's condition—no matter how subtle—because part of the nurse's responsibility is to notice changes that may indicate a worsening of the patient's condition and intervene before the situation becomes critical.

Prior to *Identifying Signs and Symptoms*, the nurse must first know what patient assessments to make. What assessments to make is dependent on the three factors previously listed:

1. The nurse's knowledge base

2. Personal characteristics of the nurse such as preconceived attitudes and self-confidence

3. The context of the individual patient situation and the type of healthcare environment: acute care, long term care, clinic, medical office, school, and other settings where nurses practice

Example Using "Identifying Signs and Symptoms" in Everyday Life

As discussed in Chapter 1, all the clinical judgment competencies used in nursing are actual thinking skills used in everyday life. There are many times throughout the day when you collect signs and symptoms of a situation and compare that data to what is normal or to what is expected in that situation. For example, you arrive home from work at 11 p.m. Your normal expectations about the condition of the house are: kitchen clean, dishes from dinner put away, quiet house, teenage children in bed, one light on in the living room to help you navigate.

One Friday evening you arrive home and find the following: kitchen is a mess with pizza boxes and remaining pizza on counter, soft drink cans in the sink, the television on, lights on in every room, and teenage children in bed.

Identifying Signs and Symptoms present in the environment this evening leads you to conclude that what took place in the home that evening was different than what normally occurs. The current situation represents signs (objective data) of a problem. To further investigate, you collect subjective information (explanation from the children) about what occurred during the evening. An investigation with application of other thinking competencies is needed prior to arriving at a conclusion about these findings.

Thinking Challenge

Provide an example of how you use the clinical judgment competency of *Identifying Signs and Symptoms* in your everyday life.

Example Using "Identifying Signs and Symptoms" in Nursing

The nurse is caring for a patient who is one day post open abdominal surgery for a ruptured appendix. When performing a nursing assessment, the nurse must collect information about signs and symptoms related to the patient's condition. As discussed earlier, using clinical forethought the nurse uses nursing knowledge to determine what signs and symptoms are expected prior to visiting the patient. Signs and symptoms to consider for this situation might include diagnostic tests, the physiology of body systems, pathophysiology of the disease, and care of the post-operative patient. Additionally, the nurse might review previous nurses' notes. Using clinical forethought to focus while *Identifying Signs and Symptoms* helps the nurse to be mindful as discussed in Chapter 1. This helps to ensure all important information related to signs and symptoms is gathered during the assessment.

Expected Clinical Picture

- Vital signs within normal limits for patient
- Relief of pain with patient-controlled analgesia
- Abdominal dressing in place, dry, and intact
- Clear, straw-colored urine in urinary drainage bag
- IV solution as ordered and running at prescribed rate
- Alert and oriented to person, place, time, and situation if this was the level of functioning prior to the surgery
- Bowel sounds faint

When you visit your patient, your assessment reveals:

- Vital signs are within patient's normal range

- The patient rates pain a 3 on a 0 to 10 scale

- The abdominal dressing is intact but there is an area of fresh blood. The patient states it was not there an hour ago

- The urine in the drainage bag is clear, straw-colored, and about 150 milliliters (emptied one hour ago)

- The IV solution and rate are as prescribed

- The patient is awake and oriented x 4 (to person, place, time, and situation)

- Bowel sounds are faint in all four quadrants

Identifying Signs and Symptoms you find that all seems well, with the exception of the fresh blood on the dressing. More investigation with application of other clinical judgment competencies is needed to make meaning of this finding.

Cognitive Guidance Tool for the Clinical Judgment Competency of "Identifying Signs and Symptoms"

COGNITIVE GUIDANCE
TOOL

This tool guides your use of the clinical judgment competency of *Identifying Signs and Symptoms*. There are many times you will use this clinical judgment competency in a variety of situations. This tool is just one example. Fill in the information or answer the questions on a piece of paper or use an electronic device as instructed by your faculty.

Gathering Information Related to Signs and Symptoms

The first step in *Identifying Signs and Symptoms* is to gather information. To gather information address each of the following:

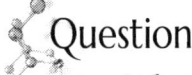
Question

What is the condition/situation/issue you are assessing?

You will use this information to determine what signs and symptoms to consider then later use that information to determine data that are out of the normal range (also called a variance). The condition/situation/issue may be a medical diagnosis such as acute asthma or a specific issue such as fever. For a medical diagnosis you may need to review the pathophysiology of that diagnosis to determine what signs and symptoms are related to that condition. The condition/situation/issue may also require identifying the signs and symptoms about a concept such as perfusion or safety.

Answer the following questions about your knowledge base related to the condition/situation/issue identified in the first question above:

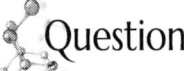
Question

What do you know about this condition/situation/issue?

Question

What do you need to review in a reference book prior to assessing the patient to identify signs and symptoms?

Question

What information will you collect and what sources will you use to gather the needed information? Here are example sources of information you can use:

- Report from the nurse on the previous shift
- The patient's medical record
    - ~ Lab results
    - ~ Previous nurse's documentation in the patient's medical record (last 24 hours)
    - ~ Other information from the medical record
- Patient self-report and other interactions with the patient
- Patient assessment conducted by the nurse
- Interprofessional team members
- Equipment in the room such as monitors, pumps, etc.

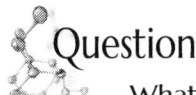

Question

What information did you glean from using the *Scanning the Environment* clinical judgment competency that can be used to collect additional signs and symptoms?

For example, if you noticed the patient has a urinary catheter in place but did not receive that information in the report from the previous nurse, you will need to consider signs and symptoms related to fluid intake, urinary output, and characteristics of urine such as color, clarity, and odor.

After you have gathered all the information, you will identify signs and symptoms. Complete Table 3.4.

TABLE 3.4

Identifying Signs and Symptoms

Data Collected	Normal or expected findings for the condition/situation/issue being assessed	Which patient data are outside of the normal range or expected findings that indicate an area of concern that needs to be addressed?

Add additional rows as needed

As you learn more about nursing, you will discover tools that are available for *Identifying Signs and Symptoms* about many specific patient care issues. For example, there are tools for assessing pain level and ones that assess a patient's risk for a fall. These tools guide you about what signs and symptoms to consider when assessing pain or the patient's risk for a fall.

As suggested by the activities of this tool, you first determine what information to collect, how to augment your knowledge as needed, and sources of information that yield the desired information. You then collect data related to the signs and symptoms you determine are important to assess related to the condition/situation/issue.

STEP 1: CLINICAL JUDGMENT COMPETENCIES

Getting the Information

ASSESSING SYSTEMATICALLY AND COMPREHENSIVELY

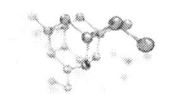

assessing systematically and comprehensively ~

making sure all information about a patient is gathered so the nurse can plan the necessary care for the patient as well as identify any potential problems that might occur or are already occurring

Definition of "Assessing Systematically and Comprehensively"

Assessing Systematically and Comprehensively means making sure all information about a patient is gathered so the nurse can plan the necessary care for the patient as well as identify any potential problems that might occur or are already occurring. The "systematically" part of the competency means a planned approach is used so the collection of data is planned and not gathered in an unorganized way that may result in missing important information. The "comprehensively" part of the competency ensures all related data are collected.

Assessing Systematically and Comprehensively helps you stay focused when gathering data. Remember the information in Chapter 1 about being mindful? It is important to remain mindful when collecting data. Collecting patient data can be stressful at times, especially if you are concerned about the patient's condition. *Assessing Systematically and Comprehensively* helps you be fully present and attentive in the moment so you do not miss any important patient information.

Data revealed when implementing the clinical judgment competencies of *Determining Important Information to Collect, Scanning the Environment,* and *Identifying Signs and Symptoms* may indicate a need for a deeper look into a specific area of concern. For example, there was no indication from the previous nurse's report that the patient was confused. However, while *Identifying Signs and Symptoms* the patient answered questions in a confused, incorrect manner. This new finding requires the nurse to further investigate. The nurse will now approach this new finding with a systematic process related to a patient's mental status to ensure relevant patient information is identified. The clinical judgment competency of *Assessing Systematically and Comprehensively* is used to ensure all related patient data are collected. The need to collect that additional information is triggered by the unexpected finding about the patient's mental status. Chapter 1 described one reason to learn clinical judgment is to deal with unexpected occurrences. This clinical judgment competency helps you do just that.

Assessing Systematically and Comprehensively is a clinical judgment competency applied to all areas of nursing practice. For example, when assessing patients, nurses use a systematic method such as a body system or a head-to-toe approach so no areas are missed. The type of patient or patient care environment does not matter; assessing systematically and comprehensively is a clinical judgment competency that must be used for all patients in the normal course of conducting a patient assessment. Additionally, any time an unexpected finding is identified, the nurse must further investigate by conducting a more in-depth, focused assessment of the affected system(s). A focused assessment means identifying information related to the unexpected finding and collecting further data that relate to that information.

The clinical judgment competency of assessing systematically and comprehensively is also used as a routine event with other nursing tasks other than patient assessment. For example, a systematic and comprehensive approach is used for data collection to prepare a report for the oncoming nurse or when notifying the primary healthcare provider such as the physician or nurse practitioner. Most nurses use a specific format for reporting patient data to ensure a comprehensive report is provided and all the important areas of information are noted. The actual format of the report is consistently used, but to collect the information that goes on that report is based on full knowledge of the clinical judgment competencies used in the "Getting the Information" step of the Caputi Clinical Judgment Framework.

Example Using "Assessing Systematically and Comprehensively" in Everyday Life

There are many times when the thinking competency of *Assessing Systematically and Comprehensively* is used in everyday life. Consider the thinking you might do to prepare to shop for a new car. The thinking you use to plan your shopping prepares you to *Assess Systematically and Comprehensively* when at the car dealership.

Because you have experience purchasing a car you realize how salespersons may distract you with features of a car in an effort to sell the vehicle. They may distract you from being mindful and keeping focused in your thinking. To prevent becoming distracted by the salesperson you make a list of important features you want in the car to avoid being persuaded to buy a car without what you desire because the salesperson focused on other features—features you are not interested in, but are meant to "wow" you into buying that particular vehicle by turning your attention away from features you want that the car does not have. Therefore, prior to visiting the first car dealership you realize the importance of identifying what you are looking for in this new car so you will not be easily distracted. You develop a list of car features you find important. To be sure you don't miss any important features you group them into categories. Your list may look something like this:

Car Assessment

Performance Features

- 4 cylinder
- 25 miles to the gallon
- Good pick-up when passing another car

Safety Features

- Backup camera
- Blind spot indicator on side mirrors
- Beeper for close contact with an object

Pleasure/Comfort Features

- Satellite radio
- Heated steering wheel
- USB port in front & back
- Smooth ride in the back seat
- Heated seats in both front seats (perhaps in the back if possible)

When you visit car dealerships you find your assessment of possible cars to purchase is controlled, without distraction from the salesperson. Your assessment is systematic and comprehensive; systematic in that you have a planned, organized approach and comprehensive meaning you are not missing any of the important features you want in this vehicle. You remain mindful during your visit to the car dealership, even if the visit becomes stressful.

Awareness of these features and a systematic approach to your assessment yield the most reliable and complete information on which to make a decision and take action.

Thinking Challenge

Provide an example of how you use the clinical judgment competency of *Assessing Systematically and Comprehensively* in your everyday life.

Example Using "Assessing Systematically and Comprehensively" in Nursing

Assessing Systematically and Comprehensively requires the ability to look beyond the obvious. For example, the patient's blood pressure is 160/90. It is obvious to the nurse the blood pressure is elevated and, for this patient, the 160/90 reading is unexpected. The nurse now starts to ask questions such as: What information is related to the blood pressure? What information do I need to collect that I will need to know when I "Make Meaning" of this new finding?

A systematic and comprehensive approach requires the nurse to further investigate by collecting additional data related to that finding. The nurse must gather sufficient data that can be used in the "Making Meaning of the Information" step to reach a reasonable conclusion. The nurse sorts through his/her nursing knowledge to determine what factors can affect a patient's blood pressure. The nurse determines factors that may affect the patient's blood pressure include level of pain, medications the patient may be receiving (or not receiving if the patient is hypertensive but an antihypertensive medication was not prescribed), pre-existing conditions the patient may have, and the stress of being in the hospital. With this knowledge the nurse assesses the patient's pain level, reviews the medications the patient is receiving, reads the patient's medical record to determine if the patient has any pre-existing conditions, and talks with the patient to determine level of stress. All this additional information as it relates to the patient's blood pressure reading is collected at this time in response to the unexpected elevated blood pressure. That additional information related to an elevated blood pressure would not have been considered if the blood pressure reading had been normal.

Assessing systematically supports the goal of assessing comprehensively; that is, when an assessment of any type is performed based on a systematic approach, that approach provides the best chance for a comprehensive assessment. Comprehensive implies a complete assessment that yields all data important to the situation. A systematic approach is used to ensure nothing important is left out of the assessment. Nurses use a systematic approach as a form of mental discipline to ensure a comprehensive data collection.

Assessing Systematically and Comprehensively relates to factors other than the patient's condition. For example, the nurse has the responsibility to keep the patient safe. The nurse assesses the patient and the patient's environment in a systematic and comprehensive manner to ensure a safe care environment. Following are some important factors to consider when ensuring a safe care environment in a systematic and comprehensive manner.

> *The nurse assesses the patient and the patient's environment in a systematic and comprehensive manner to ensure a safe care environment.*

Safety Assessment

Patient

- Positioning
- Nonslip socks
- Tubes
- Equipment
- Other factors to consider for this particular patient:

_____

_____

_____

Environment

- Clutter
- Height of the bed
- Call light within reach
- Gloves available
- Sink for hand hygiene and hand sanitizer
- Sharps container
- Other factors for this particular healthcare setting/unit:

_____

_____

_____

There are many important safety factors to consider with each patient and the patient's environment. Using a list that organizes many of these factors provides a comprehensive safety assessment. Organizing the factors into groups then referencing each of these groups as a way to systematically organize your thinking helps ensure a comprehensive assessment. Repeated use of this tool helps your thinking become automatic. Revise this list by adding more items as you learn more about nursing or to customize the tool for a specific care environment, such as for the intensive care unit or for care in the patient's home.

Cognitive Guidance Tool for the Clinical Judgment Competency of "Assessing Systematically and Comprehensively"

COGNITIVE GUIDANCE TOOL

This tool guides your use of the clinical judgment competency *Assessing Systematically and Comprehensively*. There are many times you will use this clinical judgment competency in a variety of situations. This tool is just one example. Fill in the information or answer the questions on a piece of paper or use an electronic device as instructed by your faculty.

Assessing Pain Systematically and Comprehensively

Nurses use many tools to ensure data collection is systematic and comprehensive for the purpose of gathering all necessary data. One example of a systematic and comprehensive approach to data collection is an assessment of a patient's pain. The International Association for the Study of Pain (IASP, n. d.) defines pain as "an unpleasant sensory and emotional experience associated with, or resembling that associate with, actual or potential tissue damage" (https://www.iasp-pain.org/resources/terminology/#pain). This definition emphasizes the need for nurses to conduct a systematic and comprehensive assessment of the patient's experience of pain.

Because pain is a subjective experience, the patient is the key source of information. There are a variety of mnemonics (memory tools) nurses use as reminders about the information they need to collect when assessing the patient's pain. Each school of nursing chooses which mnemonic to teach. The one you are learning may be somewhat different than the one presented here. The variation presented here is just one example.

The mnemonic "OPQRSTUV" is used for the assessment of the symptoms of pain (Gélinas, 2018; Haslam, 2019; Sawhney & Martelli, 2019). The mnemonic, as well as others you may be learning, support a systematic and comprehensive assessment. You will also learn about different tools for assessing pain in different types of patient populations. For example, there are different tools for infants and persons with cognitive impairment who are unable to verbally report their symptoms.

The tool presented in Table 3.5 guides your thinking to ensure a systematic and comprehensive approach to data collection about the pain the patient is experiencing. The tool gathers information about the characteristics of pain that are important to consider when "Making Meaning of the Information."

This tool is used to systematically and comprehensively collect both subjective data (symptoms) and objective data (signs). The patient's report about pain characteristics is subjective data. Objective data include the patient's body position and vital signs that are affected by pain.

TABLE 3.5

Assessing Systematically and Comprehensively

Pain Assessment Component	Data Collection
O ~ Onset	When did the pain start?
P ~ Palliation/Provocation	What makes the pain better? Worse?
Q ~ Quality	What does the pain feel like (sharp, dull, stabbing, burning)?
R ~ Region/Radiation	Where is your pain? Does it radiate/move anywhere else?
S ~ Severity	Rate your pain on a numeric rating scale (NRS) 0 to 10, with 0 being no pain and 10 being the worst pain possible (rate at rest and with activity)
T ~ Timing	Is the pain constant or intermittent? How long does it last?
U ~ Understanding	What do you believe is causing the pain? How is the pain impacting you? Your family? The patient's perception of pain and what the pain means to the patient.
V ~ Value	What is an acceptable level for this pain (NRS 0-10)? Any other symptoms related to the pain? Anything else you would like to say about your pain?
Other Factors	Explore other factors which may influence the pain response (culture, past pain experiences, medical history related to pain)
Pain Behaviors (verbal and non-verbal pain indicators)	Verbal expressions of pain. Non-verbal indicators of pain (facial features, body, muscle tension, moaning, crying)
Affective Responses	Signs of anxiety, depression, patterns of interacting with others, affect of pain on ability to perform daily activities, adaptive mechanism to cope with the pain

TABLE 3.5 (continued)

Assessing Systematically and Comprehensively

Pain Assessment Component	Data Collection
Medications	Medication and dose the patient is taking for pain
	Frequency taking the medication
	Patient's pain score prior to receiving the medication and pain relief score 30 minutes after receiving the medication
	The patient's evaluation/perception of the effectiveness of the medication
	Any side effects or effects the patient is experiencing
Non-Medication Relief Measures	What non-medication relief measures are provided to the patient (heat/cold application, positioning, relaxation, distraction, acupuncture, other)?
	Patient's evaluation of the effectiveness of the relief measures
Other Data	Note additional important information about the patient and the patient's pain not included in the above
	Note physiologic responses such as vital signs, perspiration, pupil size, nausea, muscle tension, anxiety

This systematic and comprehensive pain assessment yields important information necessary for planning the patient's care. This is an example of a tool focused on one area of nursing care. As you learn about nursing related to many other patient care issues, you will discover there are many established tools to ensure you engage in a systematic and comprehensive assessment. You can also develop your own tools to help you remember what information to gather to achieve a systematic and comprehensive assessment. The more you use developed tools, the more autonomous your assessments become. Eventually, you will no longer need to reference tools such as these. That is, with practice your thinking will become automatic and self-directed. That is the goal—becoming a self-directed thinker!

STEP 1: CLINICAL JUDGMENT COMPETENCIES

Getting the Information

ENSURING ACCURATE INFORMATION

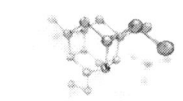

ensuring accurate information ~

verifying that collected information is accurate

Definition of "Ensuring Accurate Information"

Ensuring Accurate Information means verifying the information collected is accurate. Accurate information is a prerequisite to sound decisions. Inaccurate information leads to poor decision making which can have devastating consequences.

All the clinical judgment competencies under the step of "Gathering the Information" produce data that are used in the next four steps of clinical judgment (Making Meaning of the Information, Determining Actions to Take, Taking Action, and Evaluating Outcomes and Your Thinking). The correctness of thinking in these later steps depends on collecting data that are accurate and true. The clinical judgment competency of *"Ensuring Accurate Information"* means the nurse who collected the data took steps to verify the data are accurate. The nurse must accurately understand and communicate information without any distortions. Collecting and communicating inaccurate information can lead to decisions that result in a patient's condition worsening. To ensure accuracy, the nurse asks questions such as:

1. How can I find out if the information is true?

2. How can I verify the data are accurate?

3. How can I check to ensure the equipment used to collect the data is operating correctly?

The nurse ensures the processes used for data collection as well as the data collected are accurate. The sources of data must be deemed reliable and the processes used to gather the data must be skillfully performed. To meet this goal, nurses must be confident in their abilities to know:

1. What data to collect

2. How to accurately collect the data

3. How to ensure the data are accurate

Example Using "Ensuring Accurate Information" in Everyday Life

Ensuring the devices/equipment used to collect data are functioning properly

You are driving on the highway. A police officer turns on the flashing lights and pulls you over. The officer states you were clocked driving 15 miles per hour above the posted speed limit. She states she used a speed gun to record your speed. It is the officer's responsibility to ensure the device is functioning properly so the data recorded are accurate.

Ensuring the data collected are accurate

Here is another example of ensuring data are accurate. As you are shopping for a new car it is important to gather accurate data about the car prior to purchase. To gather accurate data, you identify sources of information that are reliable. Sources of information include:

- Manufacturer's website
- Vehicle rating websites
- Acquaintances who own a similar make and model
- If this is a used car, a reliable website that gives the history of the car's accidents

Based on information gleaned from these reliable sources of accurate information you are prepared to visit car dealerships. This information is used to balance the information provided by other sources of information that may be less reliable in accuracy such as the salesperson who has a personal interest in selling the car.

Thinking Challenge

Provide an example of how you use the clinical judgment competency of *Ensuring Accurate Information* in your everyday life.

Example Using "Ensuring Accurate Information" in Nursing

There are many areas related to patient care that require use of the clinical judgment competency of *Ensuring Accurate Information*. Nurses review patient laboratory results that measure various body functions. If a laboratory result is out of range and reaches a critical level (a level that indicates the patient is in serious condition), another specimen may be collected and tested. The results of the second specimen tested are compared to the first to ensure the results are accurate. Reasons for the repeat testing are to determine if the specimen was accurately collected, if the instrument processing the specimen is functioning correctly, or if the processing of the specimen was accurately implemented all of which are needed to be accurate to yield reliable data.

Another example of ensuring the information nurses collect is accurate is selection of a blood pressure cuff. The blood pressure cuff is selected based on the size of the patient's arm. The wrong size cuff can yield inaccurate readings. This is an example of ensuring the equipment that is used yields correct patient information.

Another important aspect of *Ensuring Accurate Information* is the source of the information. As nurses care for patients, they must identify and locate reliable sources of accurate information. Some of the sources of reliable information include:

- Professional online websites for sources of current information
- The experiences of other nurses with whom you are working
- Your nursing teacher/preceptor
- Textbooks and other reference materials with a current copyright date

Finally, the nurse assesses the patient's ability to provide accurate information. If the patient is experiencing confusion or dementia, or is under the influence of an opioid medication, the patient may not be an accurate source of information. Ensuring the patient is a reliable historian is an important aspect of *Ensuring Accurate Information*.

COGNITIVE GUIDANCE TOOL

Cognitive Guidance Tool for the Clinical Judgment Competency of "Ensuring Accurate Information"

Any information gathered about patients or a problem in the healthcare setting must be accurate. Using inaccurate information can lead to poor decisions and poor patient outcomes. For example, using the wrong size blood pressure cuff can result in a wrong blood pressure reading. A patient's blood pressure medication may be given or held based on that inaccurate reading. It is critical that all data are accurate.

This tool guides your use of the clinical judgment competency of *Ensuring Accurate Information*. There are many times you will use this clinical judgment competency in a variety of situations. This tool is just one example. Fill in the information or answer the questions on a piece of paper or use an electronic device as instructed by your faculty.

Ensuring Equipment is Yielding Accurate Information

Nurses use many types of equipment to gather patient data. Ensuring the equipment is right for the job and that the equipment is working correctly gives the nurse confidence in the accuracy of the data collected.

Conduct an inventory of the equipment on the clinical unit used to collect and measure patient data. Add that equipment to the left column of Table 3.6. Some equipment is already listed. In the right column explain how you will ensure the equipment is what is needed for the patient and/or the equipment is functioning properly.

TABLE 3.6

Ensuring the Accuracy of Equipment Used to Collect Patient Data

Equipment used to collect patient data	How you will ensure you are using the right piece of equipment, the equipment is functioning properly, you are using the equipment correctly, and the equipment reports the information accurately
Electronic thermometer	
Blood pressure cuff	
Blood glucose meter	
Pulse oximeter	
Add more equipment present on the clinical unit	

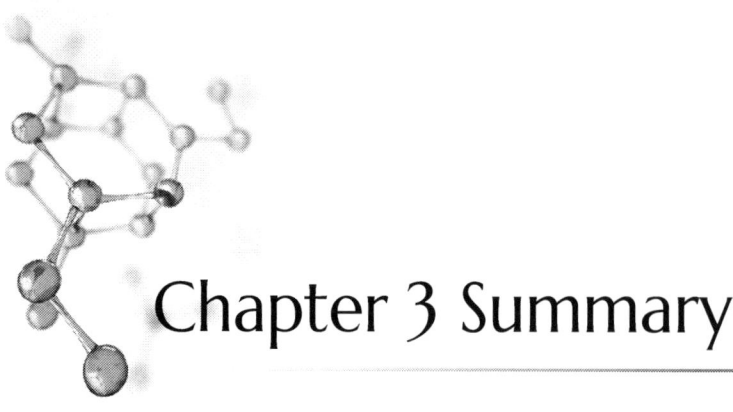

Chapter 3 Summary

This chapter covered...

Step 1 of the Caputi Clinical Judgment Framework:
"GETTING THE INFORMATION"

Also explained in this chapter were the five clinical judgment competencies of "Getting the Information:"

1. Determining Important Information to Collect

2. Scanning the Environment

3. Identifying Signs and Symptoms

4. Assessing Systematically and Comprehensively

5. Ensuring Accurate Information

Table 3.7 was first presented in Chapter 2, and also at the beginning of this chapter. This table demonstrates that the first step of the Caputi Clinical Judgment Framework aligns with the Clinical Judgment Measurement Model of the NCLEX's cognitive process of "Recognize Cues."

"Getting the Information" also aligns with the "Assessing" step of the nursing process. This demonstrates how "Getting the Information" supports the thinking needed for both the NCSBN's "Recognize Cues" cognitive process and the "Assessing" step of the nursing process. It's all about the thinking!

TABLE 3.7

Alignment of the NCSBN Clinical Judgment Measurement Model, the Caputi Clinical Judgment Framework, and the Steps of the Nursing Process

The Cognitive Processes of the NCSBN Clinical Judgment Measurement Model (Next Generation NCLEX)	Major Steps in the Caputi Clinical Judgment Framework	Steps of the Nursing Process
1. Recognize Cues	Getting the Information	Assessing
2. Analyze Cues	Making Meaning of the Information	Diagnosing
3. Prioritize Hypotheses	Determining Actions to Take	Planning
4. Generate Solutions	Determining Actions to Take	Planning
5. Take Actions	Taking Action	Implementing
6. Evaluate Outcomes	Evaluating Outcomes and Your Thinking	Evaluating

Both the Clinical Judgment Measurement Model of the NCLEX and the nursing process list steps that are general. These steps do not provide the specific thinking (clinical judgment competencies) required with each step. The Caputi Clinical Judgment Framework fills in those missing pieces. These five clinical judgment competencies form the basis for thinking that will be measured on the NCLEX exam that is determining the candidate's ability to engage in the cognitive process of "Recognize Cues." Success on the NCLEX requires being able to think using these very detailed thinking competencies so you can "Recognize Cues."

These clinical judgment competencies also represent the type of thinking you use when implementing the "Assessing" step of the nursing process. To ensure your thinking supports both the "Recognize Cues" cognitive process and the "Assessing" step of the nursing process, you must drill down to the detail provided by learning these five clinical judgment competencies.

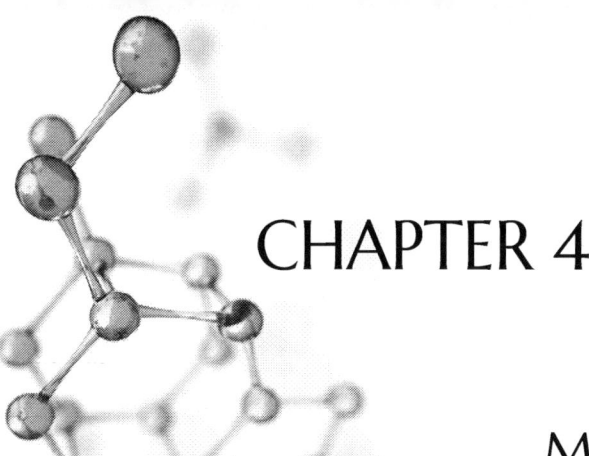

CHAPTER 4

Step 2: Making Meaning of the Information
(NCLEX®~Analyze Cues)

TABLE 4.1

The Caputi Clinical Judgment Framework: Step 2

Major Steps in the Caputi Clinical Judgment Framework	The Caputi Clinical Judgment Competencies
STEP 1 ~ Getting the Information	• Determining important information to collect • Scanning the environment • Identifying signs and symptoms • Assessing systematically and comprehensively • Ensuring accurate information
STEP 2 ~ Making Meaning of the Information	• Clustering related information • Identifying assumptions • Recognizing inconsistencies • Distinguishing relevant from irrelevant information • Judging how much ambiguity is acceptable • Comparing and contrasting • Predicting potential complications • Collaborating with healthcare team members • Determining patient care needs/healthcare environment issues
STEP 3 ~ Determining Actions to Take	• Selecting interventions • Managing potential complications • Setting priorities
STEP 4 ~ Taking Action	• Determining how to implement the planned interventions • Delegating • Communicating • Teaching others
STEP 5 ~ Evaluating Outcomes and Your Thinking	• Evaluating data • Evaluating and correcting thinking

Chapter Note

If you are reading this chapter without first reading Chapter 3, please return to the first part of Chapter 3 and read the following sections:

- How the Content is Presented
- Using the Clinical Judgment Competencies

As shown in Table 4.1, this chapter presents the clinical judgment competencies under Step 2: "Making Meaning of the Information" of the Caputi Clinical Judgment Framework. This step is all about making sense of the information collected in Step 1.

Table 4.2 demonstrates how the "Making Meaning of the Information" step aligns with the NCSBN's cognitive process of "Analyze Cues" (NCSBN, 2019) and the Diagnosing step of the nursing process. **Remember,** the Caputi Clinical Judgment Framework is the detailed thinking used with the six cognitive processes that are tested on the Next Generation NCLEX and the thinking behind the nursing process. This is demonstrated with Tables 4.2 and 4.3.

TABLE 4.2

Alignment of the NCSBN Clinical Judgment Measurement Model, the Caputi Clinical Judgment Framework, and the Steps of the Nursing Process

The Cognitive Processes of the NCSBN Clinical Judgment Measurement Model (Next Generation NCLEX)	Major Steps in the Caputi Clinical Judgment Framework	Steps of the Nursing Process
1. Recognize Cues	Getting the Information	Assessing
2. Analyze Cues	Making Meaning of the Information	Diagnosing
3. Prioritize Hypotheses	Determining Actions to Take	Planning
4. Generate Solutions	Determining Actions to Take	Planning
5. Take Actions	Taking Action	Implementing
6. Evaluate Outcomes	Evaluating Outcomes and Your Thinking	Evaluating

CHAPTER 4 ■ Step 2: Making Meaning of the Information (NCLEX® ~ Analyze Cues)

Table 4.3 lists the specific thinking processes (clinical judgment competencies) that are needed to be skillful at implementing the "Analyze Cues" cognitive process of the NCSBN's Clinical Judgment Measurement Model. It will be difficult to "Analyze Cues" without learning the detailed thinking that supports that type of thinking.

TABLE 4.3

Analyze Cues (Next Gen NCLEX Cognitive Process) Aligned to the Clinical Judgment Competencies of "Making Meaning of the Information"

NCSBN's Clinical Judgment Measurement Model Cognitive Process	Clinical Judgment Competencies in Caputi's "Making Meaning of the Information" Step
Analyze Cues	Clustering related information
	Identifying assumptions
	Recognizing inconsistencies
	Distinguishing relevant from irrelevant information
	Judging how much ambiguity is acceptable
	Comparing and contrasting
	Predicting potential complications
	Collaborating with healthcare team members
	Determining patient care needs/healthcare environment issues

The thinking skills used in the Step 1: "Getting the Information" yield information about the individual patient situation or a situation in the healthcare environment. Step 2: "Making Meaning of the Information" requires you to analyze the data to make sense of all the data collected. In the "Making Meaning of the Information" step, once you sort through the information and analyze the information you collected, you use the results of your analysis in Step 3: "Determining Actions to Take."

The clinical judgment competencies used when "Making Meaning of the Information" help answer questions such as:

- What do the data mean?

- How should the data be interpreted for this patient or situation?

- What are the most important data to consider?

- Is there enough data to determine patient care needs or how to address a healthcare environment issue or do I need to collect more information?

Therefore, in the "Making Meaning of the Information" step your goal is to:

- Process the information you collected related to the patient and/or the healthcare environment issue.

- Analyze that data to arrive at a clear, accurate understanding of the situation.

- Determine if there is any information missing.

- Have a good understanding of the situation that will be used in Step 3: "Determining Actions to Take."

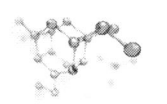

situational awareness ~

to accurately:

1) perceive clearly the meaning of the situation;

2) understand the meaning of what is happening in the situation;

3) predict what may happen in the situation

Accurate analysis of the data is critical if you are to make good decisions. Good decisions are the foundation for quality, safe, effective nursing care. An overall term that reflects the thinking used in Step 2: "Making Meaning of the Information" is **situational awareness** (White, et al., 2021). Situational awareness means the nurse is able to accurately:

1. Perceive clearly the meaning of the situation

2. Understand the meaning of what is happening in the situation

3. Predict what may happen in the situation

All three factors of situational awareness are critical for quality, safe patient care. The nurse who is situationally aware is able to determine how quickly nursing interventions must be implemented. This is known as time to task (Shinnick & Woo, 2018).

Once the nurse is aware of a patient situation, how quickly should the nurse take action? Some nursing actions can wait (as will be discussed under Setting Priorities in Step 3). However, some situations need immediate action (the patient has no pulse; the patient is demonstrating signs of sepsis [severe infection]).

Determining time to task is dependent on correctly using the 9 clinical judgment competencies of Step 2: "Making Meaning of the Information." Accurate situational awareness can only occur if the student is well-educated and has engaged in frequent use of clinical judgment.

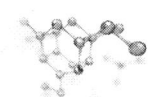

time to task ~

determining how quickly nursing interventions must be implemented

STEP 2: CLINICAL JUDGMENT COMPETENCIES

Making Meaning of the Information

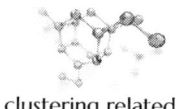

clustering related information ~

grouping together information with a common theme (such as related signs and symptoms, laboratory or diagnostic study results, pre-existing conditions, and other assessment data) in order to find meaning

CLUSTERING RELATED INFORMATION

Definition of "Clustering Related Information"

Clustering related information refers to grouping together information with a common theme. This is the process used when formulating nursing diagnoses and when identifying patient problems or concerns. Related signs and symptoms and other information such as laboratory or diagnostic study results, pre-existing conditions, and other assessment data are clustered together to make the information meaningful. Clustering related information is foundational to determining the patient's care needs, identify changes in the patient's condition, and determine appropriate responses to prevent a worsening condition that can lead to patient deterioration.

The clinical judgment competency of clustering related information also pertains to solving workplace issues and problems. Identification of information that demonstrates the cause of a workplace issue helps direct the nurse to possible solutions.

Example Using "Clustering Related Information" in Everyday Life

When an issue is identified, related information helps to provide a clearer picture of what the exact problem is. A clear picture is needed to make sound decisions about what actions to take. If all the related data are not clustered together, important information is missing and a faulty decision may occur.

For example, when organizing a large family gathering, the event planner decided to look at the weather forecast to consider holding the event outside. The weather forecast for the day was:

- Sunny conditions
- Temperature of 80 degrees
- Dew point of 72 degrees
- Winds 20 miles per hour with gusts up to 35 miles per hour
- UV index: 1 (low)
- Cloud cover: 25%
- Visibility: 10 miles

With these weather details revealing a sunny, clear, warm day, the planner decided to hold the event outside. The planner ordered a tent with tables and chairs for eating the meal, large tables to hold dining supplies, and lawn game equipment. Over 50 people were invited to the event.

The event was held and proved to be a disaster. The planner did not cluster all related information prior to making decisions, but only considered some of the data. Data the planner did not consider when reviewing the weather forecast included two important elements: dew point and wind. The dew point that day was 72 degrees, which means the air was so saturated with moisture that attendees were extremely uncomfortable. The winds were sustained at 20 miles an hour with gusts up to 35 miles an hour at times throughout the afternoon. The tent was blown over and everything on the tables that was not weighted down was blown away. It was a very unpleasant event.

The planner failed to cluster all the related information prior to making the decision about the event. When *Clustering Related Information*, all information relevant to a situation must be collected which is why the clinical judgment competencies of *Determining Important Information to Collect* and *Assessing Systematically and Comprehensively* are so important. But when analyzing the information collected with those clinical judgment competencies, the person must be certain to include all information that relates to the situation to form a complete and accurate picture prior to making a decision. The event planner failed to include two important pieces of information (dew point and wind speed) although that information was available.

All relevant data are clustered together and considered as a whole prior to making a decision. The event planner did not cluster all important information prior to making the decision to hold the event outside and this resulted in negative consequences. In this situation, the event planner only chose some pieces of information to cluster to make a decision. Although the event planner was aware of all the data, other important pieces of information were not clustered together to inform a decision based on how all those pieces related to each other.

A person's ability to think skillfully determines whether the person is able to cluster the relevant data for a given situation. In this situation relevant information included the chance of rain, wind velocity, dew point for comfort when outdoors, and temperature. This same information can be used to make other decisions about the same event. For example, if the person is deciding to take an umbrella on the walk to the event, only two pieces of information are necessary; chance of precipitation and wind velocity. All the information is available, but the individual making the decision must select and cluster the information relevant to the decision that is being made.

> A person's ability to think skillfully determines whether the person is able to cluster the relevant data for a given situation.

> Nurses use Clustering Related Information to determine which data to cluster to see the "bigger picture" for a particular patient by determining how all those pieces fit together; in doing so, the nurse sees the patient as an individual. Patient care is situation-based care addressing the individual patient's needs.

Nurses use *Clustering Related Information* to determine which data to cluster to see the "bigger picture" for a particular patient by determining how all those pieces fit together; in doing so, the nurse sees the patient as an individual. Patient care is situation-based care addressing the individual patient's needs. This is the clinical judgment thinking that takes place to identify a patient problem, issue, or concern. When the nurse skillfully puts together all related information, the patient care needs become clear. This "bigger picture" look is then used when implementing some of the other clinical judgment competencies of Step 2 such as *Collaborating with Healthcare Team Members* and *Determining Patient Care Needs/Healthcare Environment Issues*. With the clustered information the nurse is able to formulate a nursing diagnosis or engage in problem identification which is the second step of the nursing process. The nursing diagnosis may be stated in formal nursing diagnosis terminology or may be stated as a patient problem, issue, concern, or concept. Whether nursing diagnosis or patient issue/problem/concern verbiage is used depends on the healthcare system.

Thinking Challenge

Provide an example of how you use the clinical judgment competency of *Clustering Related Information* in your everyday life.

Example Using "Clustering Related Information" in Nursing

The nurse reviewing the patient's plan of care notes the primary healthcare provider is to be notified if the patient's temperature is above 102 degrees Fahrenheit (38.8 degrees Celsius). The nursing assistant reports a temperature of 103 degrees F (39.4 degrees C). Before calling the primary healthcare provider, the nurse knows other information is important to gather that relates to an elevated temperature. The related information is clustered together with the single piece of information—the temperature—to make meaning of the elevated temperature. Other information the nurse collects that relates to, and will be clustered with, the temperature includes:

- White blood cell count from the morning's complete blood count (CBC) report

- Previous temperatures and how the 103 (39.4) degree reading compares; this is known as looking at the "trend"

- Blood pressure, heart rate, and respiratory rate that may indicate further problems

- Medications prescribed such as antibiotics and antipyretic agents

Clustering this information related to the elevated temperature reading is necessary to provide a complete picture of the elevated temperature when reporting to the primary healthcare provider. All the related information will be considered when making a decision about further interventions. Competency in using the clinical judgment competency of *Clustering Related Information* depends on the nurse's knowledge and ability to identify information related to the situation at hand.

Cognitive Guidance Tool for the Clinical Judgment Competency of "Clustering Related Information"

One of the most important responsibilities of a nurse is to keep the patient safe. Safety is a very important concept that has many dimensions. There are observable factors to assess such as environmental conditions related to cluttered walkways or water on the floor. However, other factors may not be so obvious. Generally, ensuring safety requires collecting a variety of types of information that are clustered together to determine threats to the patient's safety.

This tool guides your use of the clinical judgment competency of *Clustering Related Information*. There are many times you will use this clinical judgment competency in a variety of situations. This tool that clusters information related to patient safety is just one example. Fill in the information or answer the questions on a piece of paper or use an electronic device as instructed by your faculty.

COGNITIVE GUIDANCE

TOOL

One of the most important responsibilities of a nurse is to keep the patient safe. Safety is a very important concept that has many dimensions.

Clustering Information Related to Patient Safety

- Age
- Language and cultural background
- Language barriers
- Other barriers to communication (airway devices, disease process, comprehension, hearing/speech/vision loss, emotional, psychological, masks/face shields, other)
- Physical strength
- Physical limitations
- Level of consciousness
- Cognitive ability (can the patient understand instructions, read signs, understand what the signs mean, etc.)
- Effects the disease process may have on safety and explain
- Effects of medications on safety specific for this patient and explain
- Type of environment (in-patient unit, long-term care, home, etc.)
- Factors in the environment that may pose a threat to safety
- Tubes
- Equipment
- Assistance available to help the patient
- Identification band on?
- Allergy band on?
- Current information on the patient board
- Call light available
- Further information or precautions you identified that are specific for this patient

The nurse considers all these factors and uses this information to plan interventions to keep the patient safe.

CHAPTER 4 ■ Step 2: Making Meaning of the Information (NCLEX® ~ Analyze Cues)

Based on the above information you collected, list the information in Table 4.4 that indicates a potential safety issue for this patient, and think about interventions to ensure safety.

TABLE 4.4

Clustered Factors Related to Safety

Factors clustered together that indicate a potential or real safety issue	What you will do to prevent harm from the identified safety issue

Add additional rows as needed

STEP 2: CLINICAL JUDGMENT COMPETENCIES

Making Meaning of the Information

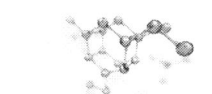

identifying assumptions ~
being aware of something that is taken for granted

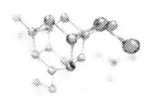

sociocentric thinking ~
adopting a self-referencing view of reality resulting from the way a person is enculturated into the various groups of society such as the family, a particular religion, or a political group

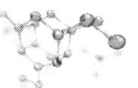

egocentric thinking ~
viewing everything in relation to oneself, an inability to see something from someone else's point of view

IDENTIFYING ASSUMPTIONS

Definition of "Identifying Assumptions"

Identifying assumptions means being aware of something that is taken for granted. What is taken for granted differs among people. Everyone's perception of the world is shaped by life experiences. Life experiences shape the lens that filters perceptions of new experiences. Because of this reality, when a person analyzes data, the data are interpreted based on that person's assumptions about many aspects of life. Assumptions are something the person takes for granted. The person assumes their way of thinking is correct. Example assumptions are that dogs and cats do not get along or drinking alcohol is inherently wrong.

Many assumptions, such as the one about alcohol, are based on sociocentric thinking. Sociocentrism refers to adopting a self-referencing view of reality. Sociocentrism results from the way a person is enculturated into the various groups of society such as the family, a particular religion, or a political group. Some beliefs may be inherent in that person—inseparable from who that person is. Unfortunately, some assumptions may even represent inherent biases. This is another connection to the goal of being mindful as discussed in Chapter 1, being aware of your assumptions.

Another influence on the development of assumptions is egocentric thinking. Egocentric thinking refers to viewing everything in relation to oneself. An example of egocentric thinking is not being able to understand why someone would make a decision that is different than the one made by oneself. Both sociocentric and egocentric thinking impedes clinical judgment.

The opinions one holds are rooted in sociocentric and egocentric thinking. This type of thinking may be acceptable when dealing with issues related to oneself; however, the individual nurse's personal opinions, thoughts, or even misunderstandings cannot be imposed on the patient.

It is critical that each nurse consider personal biases that may arise from sociocentric and egocentric thinking that are brought to the practice setting. Nurses do not intentionally apply negative assumptions in a patient situation. However, remember, a patient may be a prisoner who committed a murder or a sex offense. Some health issues such as alcoholism or other addiction are processed in many ways by the public. These situations may affect the nurse's opinion of the patient. Other areas of life such as a patient's religion, race, or sexual orientation may be different from that of the nurse. Nurses may not have much experience with some of these aspects of a patient's life or lifestyle and may make assumptions that interfere with quality care.

It is important for nurses to identify any assumptions they have about a patient's circumstances and recognize there is no place for personal opinions and biases in nursing. Nurses must recognize that the rights of patients come before the beliefs of the nurse. **Nurses are non-judgmental** and must remain non-judgmental when engaging in clinical judgment.

Nurses are non-judgmental and must remain non-judgmental when engaging in clinical judgment.

Identifying your own assumptions is critical for you to be able to seek the truth about a situation even if what you find is contrary to your own lifestyle and beliefs. Your ability to identify assumptions is rooted in being receptive to other views and sensitive to your own biases (Rubenfeld & Scheffer, 2015). Not being able to sort through assumptions and biases that may influence your thinking can result in unequal or unfair treatment of patients and others with whom you work.

Example Using "Identifying Assumptions" in Everyday Life

Assumptions people hold are not always obvious. Some not so obvious assumptions are those commonly held about the elderly. Examples include assuming all elderly people over the age of 70 are "slow" in their thinking; or that most people over the age of 80 live in long-term care facilities. It is important to recognize any possible assumptions held that lack a basis in fact. Nursing care is based on facts not assumptions.

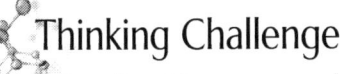

Thinking Challenge

Provide an example of how you use the clinical judgment competency of *Identifying Assumptions* in your everyday life.

Example Using "Identifying Assumptions" in Nursing

There are many situations in nursing that trigger an emotional response for the nurse. Part of the nurse's assessment is to ask patients if they feel safe at home. A negative answer may indicate possible domestic abuse. Further discussion with the patient may reveal domestic abuse has been an issue for many years for that patient. A commonly held assumption in situations of abuse and particularly long-term abuse, is that the abused has the option to leave the relationship but chooses not to leave. It is believed that if the person doesn't leave, they have accepted the abusive relationship and are willing to live a life of abuse. Such misbeliefs can foster a lack of empathy from the nurse. The ill-informed nurse will ask, "Why doesn't the person just leave?"

Once the nurse is educated in domestic abuse it becomes very apparent why the victim does not "just leave." At that point the false assumption that anyone being abused has the option to "just leave" is often dispelled. However, prior to enlightenment on the subject of domestic abuse, it is imperative nurses monitor their own beliefs and not let false assumptions interfere with quality care.

COGNITIVE GUIDANCE TOOL

Cognitive Guidance Tool for the Clinical Judgment Competency of "Identifying Assumptions"

It is necessary to identify assumptions that may interfere with the care of a patient. After receiving information about a patient and prior to visiting the patient it is helpful for the nurse to be mindful of any assumptions being made.

This tool guides your use of the clinical judgment competency of *Identifying Assumptions*. There are many times you will use this clinical judgment competency in a variety of situations. This tool that helps you identify assumptions is just one example. Fill in the information or answer the questions on a piece of paper or use an electronic device as instructed by your faculty.

Identifying Assumptions Prior to Visiting the Patient

Review the information you received from the nurse about your patient. Prior to visiting your patient, complete Table 4.5.

TABLE 4.5

Identifying Assumptions

Information about this patient	What I know about this information	Assumptions about the patient I can make based on this information
Age		
Gender identity		
Current relationship status		
Ethnocultural background		
Primary language		
Religion/spirituality		
Developmental level		
Current occupation/ employment status		
Socioeconomic status		
Type of health insurance		
Emergency code status		
Patient's expressed priorities/concerns		
Other information unique to this patient		

Now visit the patient. Ensuring sensitivity, during your conversation gather data from the patient about each of the factors listed in the table. Based on the new information complete Table 4.6.

TABLE 4.6
Challenging Assumptions

Information I collected from this patient about each factor	Identify differences from your assumptions prior to visiting the patient to what you learned while visiting the patient
Age	
Gender identity	
Current relationship status	
Ethnocultural background	
Primary language	
Developmental level	
Religion/spirituality	
Current occupation/employment status	
Socioeconomic status	
Emergency code status	
Patient's expressed priorities/concerns	
Other information unique to this patient	

Explain...
Explain the results of your analysis of assumptions.

Explain...
Talk about how those assumptions might influence the care you provide.

Explain...
Explain what you learned from this activity.

STEP 2: Making Meaning of the Information

CLINICAL JUDGMENT COMPETENCIES

RECOGNIZING INCONSISTENCIES

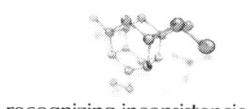

recognizing inconsistencies ~
identifying information that lacks harmony or agreement

Definition of "Recognizing Inconsistencies"

Recognizing inconsistencies refers to identifying information that lacks harmony or agreement. The data should go together in a situation, but they do not. For example, an occasional inconsistency occurring in nature is when it rains while the sun is out. The commonly held opinion is that when it is raining the sun is not shining. The two phenomena lack harmony; they should not co-exist.

The beginning point of the Caputi Clinical Judgment Framework is "Getting the Information." This aligns to the assessing step in the nursing process. As discussed in Chapter 3, when assessing ("Getting the Information") both subjective and objective data are collected. In Step 2 "Making Meaning of the Information," the data are reviewed and the nurse identifies inconsistencies between the two types of data that may indicate additional problems that are not readily apparent. Consider situations where subjective data indicate one issue, but the objective data do not support the presence of that issue. For example, the patient states he feels he is "burning up" and feels he must have a high fever. The nurse takes the patient's temperature which is 99.0 degrees Fahrenheit (37.2 degrees Celsius). These two pieces of information are inconsistent.

This is also true when gathering information about the healthcare environment. For example, a nursing assistant is responsible for taking and recording vital signs for 10 patients. Within 20 minutes after starting this task the nursing assistant states he has taken all the patients' vital signs and they are all recorded. The nurse would suspect a possible inconsistency with that information because the amount of time in which the vital signs were taken and recorded is inconsistent with the time expected to complete the task.

Example Using "Recognizing Inconsistencies" in Everyday Life

Upon rising in the morning, it is common for people to exercise. A runner looks at her phone to review the weather prediction for the next hour to determine if she should run outside or use the treadmill in her apartment. The weather app on her phone indicates rain with a chance of thunderstorms currently and for the next two hours. A look outside shows sunny skies. The information from these two sources is inconsistent. The runner is now faced with the decision about which is correct. Is the application on the phone wrong and the weather will be dry for a 45-minute run? Or, in the next 45 minutes will rain move in and she will be outside when the rain, or worse yet, a thunderstorm arrives?

This situation is an example of collecting data and identifying inconsistencies. Dealing with the issue and making a decision requires the use of other clinical judgment competencies such as *Judging How Much Ambiguity is Acceptable* (Did the app give a percentage about the chance of rain? If so, is 50% or less an acceptable number to venture running outside?). Or, perhaps she will use the clinical judgment competencies of *Predicting and Managing Potential Complications* should she decide to run outside and it begins to storm. What is the chance of a storm rather than just rain, and if a storm occurs how will that potential complication be managed?

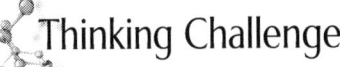

Thinking Challenge

Provide an example of how you use the clinical judgment competency of *Recognizing Inconsistencies* in your everyday life.

Example Using "Recognizing Inconsistencies" in Nursing

In addition to the above example about the nursing assistant taking vital signs, here is another example when a nurse may need to use the clinical judgment competency of *Recognizing Inconsistencies*. When completing an admission database on a 23-year-old female patient, the nurse notes the patient is 5 feet 8 inches tall, thin, pale, and weighs 103 pounds. The patient denies a history of psychological problems, eating disorders, or gastrointestinal pathology. She states she is very busy with her career and school, but is able to eat three complete meals a day. She also eats an occasional between-meal snack. She states she is fortunate she is physically active because that helps control her body weight.

Blood studies reveal a hemoglobin of 9.8g/dL (normal is 13.5 to 17.5 g/dL) and a total serum protein of 4.8 g/dL (normal is 6.3-7.9 g/dL). Hemoglobin and protein levels are indicators of nutritional status. These low values can indicate poor food intake. The subjective and objective information are inconsistent and might indicate a possible eating disorder.

COGNITIVE GUIDANCE TOOL

Cognitive Guidance Tool for the Clinical Judgment Competency of "Recognizing Inconsistencies"

The nurse analyzes information collected during the "Getting the Information" step. Inconsistencies must be sorted out to achieve a clear picture about what is happening with the patient. Practice sorting out inconsistent information will help you engage in better clinical judgment.

This tool guides your use of the clinical judgment competency of *Recognizing Inconsistencies*. There are many times you will use this clinical judgment competency in a variety of situations. This tool is just one example. Fill in the information or answer the questions on a piece of paper or use an electronic device as instructed by your faculty.

An Approach for Recognizing Inconsistencies in a Patient Situation

As nurses work with patients, they are constantly comparing patient information to what is expected based on:

- The nurse's level of knowledge
- Agency guidelines
- Evidence-based practice standards

Often there appears to be inconsistencies between the patient's presentation and that which is expected based on standard protocol. Two reasons for variances are:

1. There is something unique about this patient that requires a change to the normal protocol or approach.
2. Something may have been missed or an error was made during data collection.

Both these reasons require further investigation. The nurse must understand any variances based on sound rationale considering each patient as unique. This is part of the thinking required in Benner's Advanced Beginner stage when using situation-based thinking, as discussed in Chapter 2. However, if something was missed or an error made, the nurse must take action to correct the situation.

CHAPTER 4 ■ Step 2: Making Meaning of the Information (NCLEX® ~ Analyze Cues) 109

Complete Table 4.7

TABLE 4.7

Recognizing Inconsistencies in a Patient Situation

1	2	3	4
What is medically prescribed and/or what are nursing interventions for this patient	Textbook expectations regarding medical orders and nursing interventions	Agency guidelines or other evidence-based sources (cite source)	Differences or variances between what is ordered or planned and what is indicated in the textbook, agency guidelines, or other sources

Add more rows as needed

*Discuss each item listed in **Column 4** of Table 4.7.*

*If there are any variances,
use Table 4.8 to explain why the variance exists
and if there are any actions the nurse must take
related to that variance.*

TABLE 4.8

Explaining Variances

Differences or variances between what is ordered or planned and what is indicated in the textbook, agency guidelines, or other sources (from column 4)	Explanation about why there is a variance and actions the nurse will take or if no action needed. Explain.

Add additional rows as needed

CLINICAL JUDGMENT COMPETENCIES

DISTINGUISHING RELEVANT FROM IRRELEVANT INFORMATION

Definition of "Distinguishing Relevant from Irrelevant Information"

Relevant information is information that bears upon or is connected to the situation or matter at hand. Relevant information is pertinent. Information that is relevant directly connects to the matter at hand; irrelevant information does not connect to the matter at hand.

In Step 1 of the Caputi Clinical Judgment Framework the nurse used the clinical judgment competency of *Determining Important Information to Collect*. There is typically a lot of information to collect when assessing a patient. Hopefully, most of that information is within normal limits and/or what is expected in the patient situation.

For example, the nurse is assessing a patient who is one day postoperative and finds all vital signs are normal (118/78; respirations of 14; temperature of 98.8; pulse of 88), the patient states his pain is controlled with the ketorolac and denies any pain at the incision, bowel sounds are present but faint, the dressing on the wound is dry, there is 240 milliliters of urine in the urinal, and the patient states he just returned from a short walk down the hall with his wife and was slow but steady with no dizziness. All the information is important; however, when assessing for the possibility of a wound infection the **relevant** data are: temperature, condition of the dressing, and lack of incisional pain. (Consider how this also relates to the clinical judgment competency of *Clustering Related Information*.)

The clinical judgment competency of *Distinguishing Relevant from Irrelevant Information* refers to the nurse deciding which information is pertinent or connects with the matter at hand. All information collected about a patient may be important for the patient's overall care, but the nurse must sort out which information is relevant to a particular problem or situation currently under consideration.

STEP 2:
Making Meaning of the Information

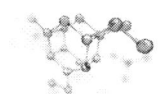

relevant information ~

pertinent information that bears upon or is connected to the situation or matter at hand

irrelevant information ~

information that does not connect to the situation or matter at hand

Example Using "Distinguishing Relevant from Irrelevant Information" in Everyday Life

Remember the situation from the clinical judgment competency of *Determining Important Information to Collect* in Chapter 3—"Getting the Information?" It went like this:

You are at the Newark, New Jersey airport scheduled on a direct, nonstop flight to the Los Angeles Airport (LAX). Your plane is delayed an hour, then another hour. Finally, the airline announces the flight has been canceled. You must now *Determine Important Information to Collect* to use to discover what flights are available that you may attempt to book for the purpose of arriving at your destination on the same day as you originally planned. There is a lot of information to sort through to determine which data are important to help meet your goal.

You immediately start to collect important information to try to arrive in Los Angeles today as intended. You collect information about:

1. Direct flights on your scheduled airline going to Los Angeles
2. Connecting flights on your scheduled airline going to Los Angeles
3. Flights on your scheduled airline going to other Los Angeles airports such as the John Wayne airport or the Ontario airport
4. Flights going to Los Angeles or a nearby airport on another airline

You have approximately 10 flights that are a possibility for you to select to meet your goal of arriving in Los Angeles this evening.

Now that you have all this important information you must *Distinguish Relevant from Irrelevant Information*. How will you do that? You'll start by determining important considerations for this thinking task. Considerations include:

1. What is the terminal and gate each of the 10 flights is leaving from? Is that terminal and gate in close proximity to you?
2. How much time is there before each of the 10 flights leave? Do you have time to get from where you are currently to the departing gate to make that flight?
3. How many other people are on the stand-by list who are trying to also get on each of those flights?
4. For flights arriving at another Los Angeles area airport, will you have ground transportation from that airport to your home?
5. If you request the airline to put you on a flight with another airline, will you have to pay a fee?

Once you determine which flights are actually feasible you have distinguished between the information which is relevant for your solution and that which is not relevant. You now have a much clearer picture of the situation and your options. You have determined only five flights will actually work for you. Now you might prioritize those flights prior to talking with an airline agent.

> ### Thinking Challenge
> Provide an example of how you use the clinical judgment competency of *Distinguishing Relevant from Irrelevant Information* in your everyday life.

Example Using "Distinguishing Relevant from Irrelevant Information" in Nursing

Remember the situation from the previous thinking skill: *Determining Important Information to Collect* that was presented in Chapter 3? It went like this:

The nurse is caring for a patient who is two days post abdominal surgery. The patient has a history of diabetes mellitus, hypertension, frequent urinary tract infection, and coronary artery disease. When visiting the patient at 0830 the patient states she is feeling a little dizzy and is somewhat confused in her thinking. The nurse decides to collect information that is important related to this patient's report of her current condition. The nurse decides to check the patient's blood sugar, blood pressure, and level of pain at the surgical site and ask about any chest discomfort. The nurse also observes the urine in the urinary drainage bag. There are many other assessments the nurse might make for this patient relative to her overall condition; however, the nurse must decide what specific information is **relevant and directly connects to the matter at hand**—the patient's report of dizziness and slight confusion.

The nurse determined what data to collect regarding the patient's report of dizziness and slight confusion based on the patient's pre-existing conditions and post-operative status. All of the pre-existing conditions might result in those symptoms. Once the data are collected the nurse must determine which of those data are relevant to the current situation of dizzy and somewhat confused. The results are as follows:

- Blood sugar of 56 (low)
- Blood pressure of 130/90 mm Hg (within patient's normal range)
- Level of pain at the surgical site: 4 on a 0 to 10 scale (pain is moderately controlled)
- Denies chest discomfort (no indication of a cardiac event)
- Urine is clear and amber color (no indication of a urinary tract infection on visual inspection)

The nurse collected important information that was specific for this patient's current issue based on the patient's history and postoperative status. The nurse did not immediately make a decision about what was causing the symptoms but collected important information specific to this patient. Once that information was collected, the nurse analyzed the data to determine which data were relevant. It appears the only piece of relevant information is the blood sugar of 56. Because a low blood sugar is often manifested by dizziness and slight confusion (*Clustering Related Information*), this relevant information leads the nurse to take action to correct the low blood sugar. In this case, using the clinical judgment competency of *Distinguishing Relevant from Irrelevant Information* resulted in an accurate determination about the source of the patient's symptoms that were then addressed with a targeted, effective intervention.

Here is another example. The nurse is caring for a patient four hours after a cardiac cauterization. While the nurse ambulates the patient the catheter insertion site in the groin begins to bleed profusely. The nurse hurriedly returns the patient to the bed, applies pressure on the bleeding site, and asks the nursing assistant to take a set of vital signs. The nursing assistant replies she would need to go to the nurses' station for a thermometer. The nurse quickly restates his request with, "Take a blood pressure and a pulse, please."

In this situation when the nursing assistant heard "a set of vital signs," she was unable to distinguish which vital signs were relevant and which were not. It was important for the nurse to intervene and ask the nursing assistant to take only the relevant vital signs to expedite the collection of data about the patient's current status and to establish a baseline should the patient's condition worsen. The clinical judgment competency of *Distinguishing Relevant from Irrelevant Information* was crucial in this time-sensitive situation. Time pressure is an environmental factor that is part of the NCSBN's Clinical Judgment Measurement Model and tested on the Next Generation NCLEX. For the patient who is bleeding, time pressure refers to quickly determining the urgency of the bleeding so proper care can be implemented to prevent a worsening condition.

Time pressure is an environmental factor that is part of the NCSBN's Clinical Judgment Measurement Model and tested on the Next Generation NCLEX.

Cognitive Guidance Tool for the Clinical Judgment Competency of "Distinguishing Relevant from Irrelevant Information"

COGNITIVE GUIDANCE TOOL

Distinguishing Relevant from Irrelevant Information is a thinking skill used throughout a nurse's time at work. The nurse often must work very quickly to distinguish what information is relevant versus that which is not. Frequent practice using this clinical judgment competency helps the student become more skillful in its use.

This tool guides your use of the clinical judgment competency of *Distinguishing Relevant from Irrelevant Information*. There are many times you will use this clinical judgment competency in a variety of situations. This tool is just one example. Fill in the information or answer the questions on a piece of paper or use an electronic device as instructed by your faculty.

Distinguishing Relevant from Irrelevant Information from All the Patient's Data

Collect the following information about your patient. This part of the tool may look familiar if you completed this tool in Chapter 3 for the clinical judgment competency of *Determining Important Information to Collect*.

1. **Patient information ~**

   - Age
   - Date of admission
   - Surgical procedure
   - Activity
   - Reason for admission
   - Diagnostic procedures
   - Diet
   - Vital signs
   - Trending of vital signs: *How have the vital signs changed from the previous reading; from the previous 24 hours?*

2. **Medications ~** *Complete for each medication prescribed.*

   - Drug prescribed
   - Therapeutic effects expected
   - Results the patient experienced
   - Reason why it was prescribed
   - Adverse effects to monitor

3. **Patient history ~**
   Review the patient's history. From the history, determine the most important data impacting this hospitalization and the patient's care.

4. Diagnostic tests ~ *Complete for each diagnostic test ordered.*
- Name of test
- Test results
- Why this test was ordered
- Trending of the results: *If the test was performed more than once, how have the results changed from the previous reading?*

Answer the following questions:

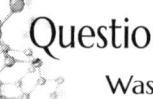
Question
Was all the information you noted important to collect for this patient?

Why? Why not?

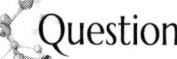
Question
Is there other information not included in the above list that you should collect? List that information and explain why it would be important to collect that information as well.

Review the data you collected to determine which data are relevant to the care of the patient on this day. All the information may be important, but your task now is to distinguish which data are relevant and how that data will influence the care you provide for this patient today.

In the left-hand column of Table 4.9 list the information you recorded that you believe are relevant data. In the right-hand column discuss why that data are relevant for the current, immediate care of this patient.

TABLE 4.9

Relevant Data for Patient Care

Data that are relevant to the patient's care today	Why those data are relevant

Add additional rows as needed

CHAPTER 4 ■ Step 2: Making Meaning of the Information (NCLEX® ~ Analyze Cues)

Remember, although all the information was important to review, only some of the data are relevant for planning care for this day.

Consider the following approach and answer the questions:

Question
Are there findings present now that were not previously apparent?

Question
Are there data that indicate a problem is developing or already present?

Question
Examine data that have changed from previous readings.

Are those changes indicative of the patient improving?

Are those data indicative of the patient's condition worsening?

Question
Are the medications working? What tells you **yes** they are working or **no** they are not working?

STEP 2: CLINICAL JUDGMENT COMPETENCIES

Making Meaning of the Information

JUDGING HOW MUCH AMBIGUITY IS ACCEPTABLE

Definition of "Judging How Much Ambiguity is Acceptable"

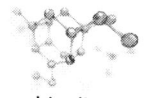

ambiguity ~

being unclear, uncertain, or vague; occurs when factors relating to a situation make applying a rule somewhat grey

Ambiguity refers to being unclear, uncertain, or vague. Life has many rules for the purpose of providing order in a society or guidelines for approaching a problem. However, there are times when a rule cannot be applied exactly as written. Ambiguity occurs when factors relating to a situation make applying the rule somewhat grey. **That is, the rule is not always strictly applied because of specific circumstances present within a given situation.** Many situations appear similar on the surface, but actually differ when all factors about each situation are carefully considered.

Consider what you learned in Chapter 2 about Dr. Benner's Novice to Expert theory. As a novice you apply all the rules you learn in the exact same way for all patients regardless of the situation. However, with learning these clinical judgment competencies you are discovering that how those rules you learned are applied really depends on the situation. You must make meaning of details related to a specific patient prior to determining exactly how, or if, to apply a rule. In this moment you move from a Novice (rule-based thinker) to an Advanced Beginner (situation-based thinker). This is a major advance in your thinking.

You must make meaning of details related to a specific patient prior to determining exactly how, or if, to apply a rule.

Dealing with situations that superficially appear similar but are somewhat different when all the details are considered requires a close look and analysis. Details about a condition that vary from patient to patient are also called "nuances." These nuances are extremely important when "Making Meaning of the Information" collected in Step 1: "Getting the Information."

When a rule is not strictly applied, it is important to use the facts about the situation to justify modification of the rule for that situation.

When variations to the norm are present in a situation, application of a rule may require some "wiggle room." That is, the situation may require accepting as "okay" information that falls outside the limits of the rule based on the details of the situation. When a rule is not strictly applied, it is important to use the facts about the situation to justify modification of the rule for that situation. It is this phenomenon that explains the commonly held belief that nursing is not black or white but grey. Grey means that rather than strict application of a rule or guideline, application of that rule or guideline "depends" on the situation. This is often what is meant when faculty ask you to "look at the bigger picture." Consider the details of the individual patient situation as you are "Making Meaning of the Information." You will become more able to think as a situation-based thinker the more nursing content you learn. Remember, thinking depends on your ability to apply clinical judgment competencies to your nursing knowledge. At this point you are just entering the Advanced Beginner Stage of thinking. The more nursing knowledge you learn the more you will be able to function as a situation-based thinker.

Example Using "Judging How Much Ambiguity is Acceptable" in Everyday Life

When driving a car and merging onto an expressway, a rule is considered. That rule is the speed limit, with the maximum and minimum limits posted. However, before deciding how much "wiggle room" there is when considering the actual rate of speed that will be driven, the driver collects data. That data may include:

- Amount of traffic
- Weather conditions
- Visibility
- Condition of the road
- Location where police officers typically park
- Number of traffic violations the driver has

After very quickly considering all the data, the driver makes a decision about what speed **above** the posted limit can be safely driven. Or, if the data reveal issues with weather or road conditions, how much **slower** to drive than the posted minimum.

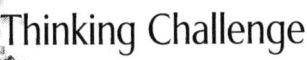
Thinking Challenge

Provide an example of how you use the clinical judgment competency of *Judging How Much Ambiguity is Acceptable* in your everyday life.

Example Using "Judging How Much Ambiguity is Acceptable" in Nursing

Early in their nursing education students learn the psychomotor skill of taking vital signs. They learn the "within normal limits" rules of vital signs. It is critical for nurses to decide how much ambiguity can be tolerated for an individual patient around the "within normal limits" of vital signs. Using this clinical judgment competency, the situation is considered and a rule applied, not in a strict sense, but in a way to determine "how much wiggle room" can be tolerated when applying the rule. For example, the nursing assistant reports to the nurse that patient #1's blood pressure is 100/60 and patient #2's blood pressure is 105/60. Based on the information the nurse obtained in the shift report, the nurse knows that he must immediately assess patient #2 (BP of 105/60), but patient's #1 (BP of 100/60) can wait. How can this be?

The nurse made this decision by looking at the individual patient context and considering other information related to each patient's condition and how that information affects the blood pressure. Patient #1's blood pressure is normal for that patient. Patient #2 is a newly admitted trauma victim under observation for internal injuries. Her blood pressure readings have not been lower than 130/85. With the blood pressure now 105/60, the nurse needs to immediately visit patient #2 to further assess the situation.

Remember: When a rule is not strictly applied (expecting a normal blood pressure), it is important to use the facts about the situation to justify modification of the rule for that situation (responding to one patient with a low blood pressure but not responding to the second patient with a low blood pressure).

When a rule is not strictly applied, it is important to use the facts about the situation to justify modification of the rule for that situation.

COGNITIVE GUIDANCE TOOL

Cognitive Guidance Tool for the Clinical Judgment Competency of "Judging How Much Ambiguity is Acceptable"

The purpose of this activity is to provide experience about how nurses think through a specific patient situation; that is, considering a rule such as "within normal limits" to a specific patient situation to determine how much wiggle room is acceptable. This assignment looks specifically at a patient's vital signs. However, the purpose of this assignment is not to teach a list of steps to memorize when considering a patient's vital signs. The purpose of the assignment is to use the clinical judgment competency of *Judging How Much Ambiguity is Acceptable* to make meaning of data to arrive at a decision based on a specific patient situation. This provides practice understanding that decisions are made not based on an individual piece of information (blood pressure is high or low), but to consider that piece of information within the whole of the patient situation. The amount of ambiguity (wiggle room) that can be tolerated requires considering that one piece of information within the total patient picture.

This tool guides your use of the clinical judgment competency of *Judging How Much Ambiguity is Acceptable*. There are many times you will use this clinical judgment competency in a variety of situations. This tool is just one example. Fill in the information or answer the questions on a piece of paper or use an electronic device as instructed by your faculty.

Judging How Much Ambiguity is Acceptable Applied to Vital Signs

This activity applies the clinical judgment competency of *Judging How Much Ambiguity is Acceptable* to make meaning of a patient's vital signs. Nurses must collect information, analyze the information, and determine the importance of the information, all within the context of the patient, then they can determine how to apply the "within normal limits" rules they learned about vital signs. The "within the context of the patient" is where the clinical judgment competency of *Judging How Much Ambiguity is Acceptable* applies. It is difficult to witness how a nurse actually uses *Judging How Much Ambiguity is Acceptable* because the thinking is completed so quickly and automatically. The purpose of this tool is to guide you through the process with a step-by-step approach that walks you through the thinking a nurse uses.

Answer the following questions:

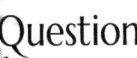
Question

What are the patient's current vital signs?

- Blood pressure
- Pulse
- Respirations
- Oxygen saturation (SpO$_2$)
- Temperature

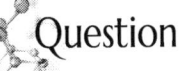
Question

What are the vital signs for the past 24 hours?

Question
What are the highs and lows for the past 24 hours?

Question
Is the patient experiencing pain?
If so, what is the patient's pain level based on a scale of 0 to 10?

Question
What is the patient's activity level?

Question
What medications is the patient taking that affect the vital signs?
Describe the effect of each medication on each of the vital signs.

Question
What medical/nursing interventions is the patient experiencing that may affect the patient's vital signs?

Question
What other factors are influencing this patient's vital sign readings?

Using the above information, address each of the following:

Question
How low can each of the readings go before you would intervene?
Give your rationale.

Question
How high can each of the readings go before you would intervene?
Give your rationale.

Question
Are the current vital signs acceptable for this patient? Explain.

CLINICAL JUDGMENT COMPETENCIES

STEP 2: Making Meaning of the Information

COMPARING AND CONTRASTING

Definition of "Comparing and Contrasting"

Comparing and contrasting involves looking at two or more situations that are similar by some common characteristic. With further study, differences among the situations emerge. Many situations appear similar on the surface but actually differ when all factors are carefully considered. These differences may not be readily apparent for those unfamiliar with the type of situations under consideration. As one becomes more familiar and has experience working with similar situations, small variances or differences become readily apparent. Small differences or variances are also known as nuances. Nuances are very slight differences or variations that can greatly affect decisions that are made.

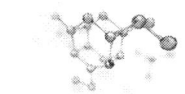

comparing and contrasting ~ looking at two or more situations that are similar by some common characteristic

Example Using "Comparing and Contrasting" in Everyday Life

Some everyday situations in which you might use *Comparing and Contrasting* include:

1. Comparing your weight to a chart

2. Comparing two or more toddlers in their ability to talk or perform a motor skill and measuring both of them against developmental milestones for that age

3. Comparing the length of one side of your hair to the other during a haircut to ensure both sides are even

4. Comparing prices for an item at three different stores

Thinking Challenge

Provide an example of how you use the clinical judgment competency of *Comparing and Contrasting* in your everyday life.

Example Using "Comparing and Contrasting" in Nursing

Using the clinical judgment competency of *Comparing and Contrasting* helps nurses recognize differences and similarities among patients or situations. These differences may be evident, or they may be very subtle. Subtle differences are called nuances. These differences or nuances make a patient situation or other nursing situation unique.

The more experience you have using *Comparing and Contrasting* with patients and situations, the more individualized patient care becomes. For example, the nurse is caring for two patients who are both one day postoperative with the same surgery. The nurse must decide how far to ambulate each patient. The nurse decides to ambulate one patient around the entire unit but decides to ambulate the second patient only to the door of the patient's room then back to the chair. Although both patients had the same surgery and are both in postop day one, the small differences, or nuances, between the two patients leads the nurse to determine the safe distance for each patient.

Comparing and Contrasting can also be applied to one patient. Remember, any time a patient has two of "something," such as two arms, always compare the one being investigated with the other that is expected to be normal. For example, the nurse looks at the patient's intravenous (IV) catheter insertion site. It appears a little swollen. The nurse is unsure if this is the normal size of the patient's arm or if it is a result of an infiltration of the IV fluid into the tissues rather than the vein. The nurse then compares the arm with the IV to the arm without an IV to determine if the swelling is a concern related to the possibility of an infiltrated IV, or if the swelling is actually not swelling but the normal size of the patient's arm.

Cognitive Guidance Tool for the Clinical Judgment Competency of "Comparing and Contrasting"

Comparing and Contrasting patients with similar situations helps the nurse discover the nuances, or small differences, among the patients. Although these differences may be small, the differences may greatly influence the decisions you make. With this cognitive guidance tool, you will practice *Comparing and Contrasting* several patient situations.

This tool guides your use of the clinical judgment competency of *Comparing and Contrasting*. There are many times you will use this clinical judgment competency in a variety of situations. This tool is just one example. Fill in the information or answer the questions on a piece of paper or use an electronic device as instructed by your faculty.

Comparing and Contrasting Three Patients for Manifestations of an Infection

For each of three patients with a diagnosis of infection, collect the following information:

Patient Information

- Age
- Number of days in hospital
- Medical diagnosis
- Pre-existing conditions
- Medications
- Activity level
- Current level of pain and pain history over the course of hospitalization
- General health status
- Nutritional status
- Hydration status
- Lifestyle including nutritional intake, tobacco use, alcohol intake, illicit substance use

Infection Present
- Type and location of infection
- Assessment and lab/diagnostics related to existing infection
- Course of treatment

Compare and contrast data for the three patients.
Answer the following questions:

Question
How are the infections the same? Different?

Question
How are the treatments the same? Different?

Question
How is each patient responding to treatment?

Question
Which individual patient factors will have the most influence on the patient's recovery from the infection?

CLINICAL JUDGMENT COMPETENCIES

PREDICTING POTENTIAL COMPLICATIONS

Definition of "Predicting Potential Complications"

A potential complication refers to the possibility that something untoward can happen in a situation. A potential complication is a happening or event that can result in an adverse reaction that aggravates or worsens the current status of the patient. Potential complications make matters worse; they move patients in the wrong direction. Rather than improving, potential complications can result in the patient not progressing or even result in the patient's condition getting worse.

Potential complications are possible for most patients receiving nursing care. Predicting potential complications is a major responsibility of the nurse and requires skillful use of clinical judgment competencies. Nurses must consider potential complications that commonly occur for all patients facing a similar situation, as well as those that might occur based on an individual patient's unique situation.

Example Using "Predicting Potential Complications" in Everyday Life

In everyday life there are often times when you predict potential complications. One example is predicting complications when weather threatens your commute home after work. The weather forecast is for heavy snow during the time you are at work. You predict you may have complications with your commute home and think ahead to determine what those possible complications might be. In nursing thinking ahead is called **clinical forethought**. In this example, potential complications may be:

- You are delayed in your car for long periods of time and run out of gas.

- You are delayed so long you miss dinner time and may grow very hungry.

- You may need to turn off the car at times to conserve gasoline and the car becomes cold.

- You may need to call for help using your cell phone.

STEP 2:
Making Meaning of the Information

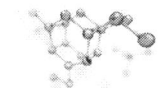

potential complication ~

the possibility that something untoward can happen in a situation resulting in an adverse reaction that aggravates or worsens the current status of a patient

Predicting potential complications is a major responsibility of the nurse and requires skillful use of clinical judgment competencies.

Once you determine the possible complications, you realize you must manage those potential complications should they occur. *Managing Potential Complications* is a clinical judgment competency included in Step 3: "Determining Actions to Take." To *Manage Potential Complications* that may occur in this example you do the following:

- Before leaving for work you fill your car's fuel tank with gas
- Pack cold weather outerwear
- Take healthy snacks and water
- Ensure your cellular phone is fully charged

You continue to monitor the weather during the day. Once the snow begins to fall at an alarmingly fast rate, you alert your supervisor who has the authority to close the business establishment early if needed. By predicting the weather may cause complications related to a safe commute home, you determine what potential complications may occur, take actions to prevent them, but also prepare to deal with those complications should they occur. Your goal is to totally prevent complications from occurring or minimize any harmful effects should a complication occur.

Thinking Challenge

Provide an example of how you use the clinical judgment competency of *Predicting Potential Complications* in your everyday life.

Example Using "Predicting Potential Complications" in Nursing

Many conditions inherently have potential complications that might occur, which is why nurses include measures focused on prevention. Nurses look at the potential complications that commonly occur with a particular problem, such as a wound becoming infected then provide frequent wound assessment for **early identification** of any signs and symptoms of infection. Nurses also institute **preventive measures** such as keeping the wound clean.

However, individual patients are also at risk for potential complications that are unique to their particular situation. Nurses must look at the total patient picture to predict potential complications that may exist on an individual basis. For example, a patient recovering from surgery with a pre-existing condition of type 2 diabetes is at risk for different potential complications than a patient with the same surgery but who does not have type 2 diabetes.

> Nurses must look at the total patient picture to predict potential complications that may exist on an individual basis.

Some potential complications carry dire consequences and require early recognition of predictable emergencies. If measures are not put into place to prevent potential complications that can quickly worsen the patient's condition, then an emergency situation is highly probable. If the patient's condition deteriorates and the patient dies, this is considered a failure to rescue situation. It is obvious that failure to rescue is extremely undesirable. Nurses must skillfully implement the clinical judgment competency of *Predicting Potential Complications* to cover all these possible scenarios.

The starting point for *Predicting Potential Complications* is to know common complications related to a patient's condition. For example, developing a blood clot in the leg from lack of movement due to bed rest or limitations on ambulation is a potential complication. Then consider individual patient differences that may result in additional concerns for that patient. A blood clot in the leg may be caused by bed rest, but further exploration of individual the patient's situation may raise your level of concern such as the patient smokes and takes birth control pills, both of which increase the risk for blood clots. A major nursing activity is to ensure preventable complications are indeed prevented.

Additional Examples

Most surgical patients are at risk for potential complications such as atelectasis and pneumonia. Interventions such as deep breathing and coughing exercises, early ambulation, and the use of an incentive spirometer are planned. However, an 18-year-old athlete in excellent physical condition who has undergone a laparoscopic appendectomy is at much less risk for these complications than a 60-year-old obese patient with a history of cigarette smoking who has undergone a colon resection. Therefore, individual factors for these two patients dictate the degree to which the preventive measures are taken. That is, the care the nurse plans to prevent complications after surgery is directly related to the individual patient situation. The 60-year-old patient may need to use the incentive spirometer more frequently than the 18-year-old athlete.

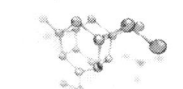

clinical forethought ~ thinking ahead to foresee any possible complications for the individual patient

Another example is a patient in your care who has a very slow pulse rate, 38 beats per minute. A potential complication is dizziness. Therefore, you ensure an alarm is in place to alert you if the patient gets out of bed alone because the dizziness may result in a fall causing harm to the patient.

In this situation the nurse is engaged in **clinical forethought**, thinking ahead to foresee any possible complications for the individual patient. Interventions to prevent complications, or to minimize the effects of complications, require use of the clinical judgment competency of *Predicting Potential Complications* to ensure the patient is safe while under your care.

COGNITIVE GUIDANCE TOOL

Cognitive Guidance Tool for the Clinical Judgment Competency of "Predicting Potential Complications"

This tool helps you *Predict Potential Complications* that may occur. It is important for you to think about potential complications because it is the nurse's responsibility to keep the patient safe. This is part of using clinical forethought. Potential complications not only relate to the patient's medical diagnosis, but also to individual factors about that patient.

Potential complications not only relate to the patient's medical diagnosis, but also to individual factors about that patient.

This tool guides your use of the clinical judgment competency of *Predicting Potential Complications*. There are many times you will use this clinical judgment competency in a variety of situations. This tool is just one example. Fill in the information or answer the questions on a piece of paper or use an electronic device as instructed by your faculty.

Analyzing Patient Information to Predict Potential Complications

Following are some commonly occurring individual factors the nurse considers that may put the patient at risk for a potential complication.

- Is there anything about this patient that leads you to believe there is a possibility the patient might fall?
- Is the patient physically weak and in need of assistance ambulating?
- Is the patient 65 years of age or older and at risk to fall?
- Is the patient cognitively impaired and not able to follow instructions?
- Does the patient have a sensory loss such as poor hearing or vision?
- Is the patient taking medications that cause dizziness or can make the patient drowsy?

*Based on your current level of nursing knowledge,
answer the following questions related to your patient.*

Question
What are you on alert for today with this patient and why?

Question
What are the important assessments to make and why?

Question
What complications may occur and why?

Question
Based on the above, what could go wrong?

Once you have learned how to *Predict Potential Complications*,
you will learn to *Manage Potential Complications* in
Step 3: "Determining Actions to Take."

STEP 2: CLINICAL JUDGMENT COMPETENCIES

Making Meaning of the Information

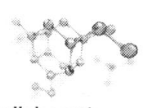

collaborating ~

to cooperatively work with others by engaging in open communication while demonstrating mutual respect and sharing decision-making

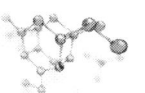

interprofessional team ~

members from various professions/groups working together to enable effective collaboration and improve health outcomes

intraprofessional team ~

members of the same profession working together to enable effective collaboration and improve health outcomes

A team approach, with all members collaborating and working together, strengthens patient care and fosters positive outcomes.

COLLABORATING WITH HEALTHCARE TEAM MEMBERS

Definition of "Collaborating with Healthcare Team Members"

Collaborating refers to cooperatively working with others. Collaboration involves engaging in open communication while demonstrating mutual respect and sharing decision-making. The goal of collaboration is to achieve a quality outcome in a given situation. Collaborating means working as a team for a mutual goal.

The resolution to a problem or approach to care seldom happens working alone; many people can be involved. When respectfully requesting information and suggestions from others, new perspectives on a situation are realized. Various approaches and solutions may be considered.

Healthcare settings are complex environments requiring the input and cooperation of many working as a team. Interprofessional team members work together and include patients, family, non-nursing health professionals, nursing health professionals, clergy, support staff, and others. Members of the same profession working together is known as an intraprofessional team. Healthcare team members engage in thinking processes when they examine delivery of care, noting compliance with standards of care and adherence to accepted protocols. Collaboration requires mutual respect, trust, and shared decision-making. A team approach, with all members collaborating and working together, strengthens patient care and fosters positive outcomes.

There are some factors to consider prior to initiating a conversation with another healthcare team member. First, you need to think through the problem or situation and determine the reason for collaborating. In doing so, organize your thoughts and have a system for communicating your concerns, including all relevant data. Healthcare facilities have adopted a system called ISBAR with many adaptations and modifications from this basic form. ISBAR is an acronym that stands for: Identify, Situation, Background, Assessment, and Recommendation. The purpose of using the ISBAR format is to ensure a systematic process for complete and accurate exchange of information when collaborating with others. ISBAR and other aspects of quality communication are addressed with the clinical judgment competency of *Communicating* in Step 4: "Taking Action."

Second, know that conflict may occur. Conflict cannot be avoided. Nurses often work in a rapidly paced environment, full of urgency and serious consequences if errors are made. In this type of environment, conflict is inevitable. Nurses in all areas of patient care must be able to maintain calm, avoid conflict, and if conflict should occur, handle it in a constructive manner. (Refer to the discussion on resiliency in Chapter 1.) These characteristics serve to promote an atmosphere that is optimal for successful and positive collaboration among healthcare team members.

Example Using "Collaborating with Healthcare Team Members" in Everyday Life

Humans are social beings and enjoy being a member of a group. As a member of a group there is much collaboration that occurs when that group is called upon to plan an event, resolve an issue, or make a decision about implementing something new. One group member's idea or perspective about the issue is just that: the idea or perspective of one person. It takes collaboration with other members of the group to ensure all relevant information is collected, to make a decision that is fair and just to all, and to ensure various perspectives are heard and considered. The goal is to achieve a group decision or plan that represents the best approach for achieving a positive outcome. Examples of groups include a religious group, sports team, or homeowners' association. When you are part of a team, you work within that team.

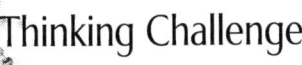

Thinking Challenge

Provide an example of how you use the clinical judgment competency of *Collaborating with Healthcare Team Members* in your everyday life.

Example Using "Collaborating with Healthcare Team Members" in Nursing

A nurse is volunteering in a free clinic. The nurse normally works on a medical unit in the local hospital. The nurse is listening to heart sounds of a 55-year-old patient. An extra sound is heard. The nurse is unsure if the sound represents a problem. The patient states he has no knowledge of any heart problem and no one has ever mentioned an extra sound when listening to his heart. The nurse can decide to not take any action since the patient has no other signs or symptoms of disease and has no history of a cardiac problem; or, the nurse can choose to collaborate with another healthcare team member. The nurse reports the finding to the nurse practitioner (NP) who operates the clinic. The NP listens to the patient's heart and decides the extra heart sound necessitates a workup. She contacts the physician to order further diagnostic testing. An echocardiogram is ordered.

As a member of the healthcare team the volunteer nurse recognized a possible problem then collaborated with the NP. It is important to note the nurse's lack of expertise in listening to heart sounds did not interfere with collaborating with others. The nurse readily shared with the NP her lack of knowledge and experience with identifying a cardiac problem based on auscultation of the patient's heart. This nurse did not hesitate to seek help because an aspect of being a professional is to know what you know and what you don't know and collaborate with other team members as needed.

COGNITIVE GUIDANCE TOOL

Cognitive Guidance Tool for the Clinical Judgment Competency of "Collaborating with Healthcare Team Members"

Working through what information you will share and with whom to share it takes careful thought. You must be mindful of the need to collaborate as you work through your day. This tool provides practice using various aspects of the clinical judgment competency of *Collaborating with Healthcare Team Members*.

This tool guides your use of the clinical judgment competency of *Collaborating with Healthcare Team Members*. There are many times you will use this clinical judgment competency in a variety of situations. This tool is just one example. Fill in the information or answer the questions on a piece of paper or use an electronic device as instructed by your faculty.

Planning to Collaborate with Members of the Healthcare Team

As you work through your day, think about aspects of patient care that require you to collaborate with other healthcare team members.

Complete Table 4.10

TABLE 4.10

Collaborating with Other Healthcare Team Members

What information will/should you share with other healthcare team members?	With which member of the healthcare team will you communicate?	What information do you expect to receive from the other team members?	What collaborative activities did you engage in?

Add more rows as needed

STEP 2: CLINICAL JUDGMENT COMPETENCIES

Making Meaning of the Information

DETERMINING PATIENT CARE NEEDS/HEALTHCARE ENVIRONMENT ISSUES

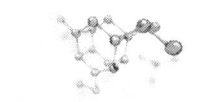

determining patient care needs/healthcare environment issues ~

accurately stating the issues, needs, problems, concerns, or anything else that requires attention

Definition of "Determining Patient Care Needs/Healthcare Environment Issues"

Determining Patient Care Needs/Healthcare Environment Issues is all about accurately stating the issues, needs, problems, concerns, or anything else that requires attention. The goal is to determine areas in need of attention that are supported by the evidence gathered in Step 1: "Getting the Information" and analyzed in Step 2: "Making Meaning of the Information." What particular conditions are present based on the evidence from the information gathered? There may be multiple issues and concerns that need to be addressed based on the analysis of the information. The goal with this clinical judgment competency is to develop a clear and accurate problem statement or nursing diagnosis (written with NANDA verbiage or as a concept problem/concern). The problem statement or diagnosis is used to "Determine Actions to Take" in Step 3 of the Caputi Clinical Judgment Framework.

For the nurse, Step 2 of the Caputi Clinical Judgment Framework is all about "Making Meaning of the Information" about the patient or about the healthcare environment. The first eight clinical judgment competencies in Step 2 work to analyze the information from Step 1: "Getting the Information." Nurses use all the clinical judgment competencies of Step 2 to make meaning then draw conclusions about what the information means. These conclusions include identifying the specific care needs of a patient or the specific issues in the healthcare environment that need to be addressed. Stating these needs and issues in a clear, accurate manner is what *Determining Patient Care Needs/ Healthcare Environment Issues* is all about.

Example Using "Determining Patient Care Needs/Healthcare Environment Issues" in Everyday Life

Most people do not make a formal problem statement for concerns that occur in everyday life. However, they do so in an informal manner. Here are common problems that can be presented as a problem statement for some of the examples of applying clinical judgment competencies in everyday life found in this text.

- Knowledge deficit related to not considering all factors when planning an outside event
- Underweight based on comparison of own current BMI to a BMI table
- Risk for driving violation related to speeding to get to work on time

Thinking Challenge

Provide an example of how you use the clinical judgment competency of *Determining Patient Care Needs/Healthcare Environment Issues* in your everyday life.

Example Using "Determining Patient Care Needs/Healthcare Environment Issues" in Nursing

The *Determining Patient Care Needs* part of this clinical judgment competency relates to formulating a nursing diagnosis or a problem statement related to a patient care need. While formulating a patient problem statement the nurse analyzes all the information collected that provide cues that verify care needs. If at any point in Step 2: "Making Meaning of the Information" the nurse determines additional information is needed to help establish the significance of cues, the nurse must return to the patient and gather that additional information.

Consider some of the information presented in this chapter to illustrate other clinical judgment competencies. Here is a listing of some patient information.

- The patient is taking an opioid analgesic and is dizzy when ambulating.
- The patient's blood pressure and hemoglobin are low.
- The patient has an IV and is using an IV pole when ambulating.

- The patient is weak from surgery the previous day.

- The patient states he is just fine and doesn't need help walking.

- The patient has type 2 diabetes.

- The patient states her pain is 7 on a 0 to 10 scale and is using patient-controlled analgesia.

After applying the many clinical judgment competencies in Step 2, the nurse formulated the following list of patient care needs:

- Potential risk for fall
  (taking an opioid for pain; dizzy when ambulating; blood pressure and hemoglobin low; ambulating with equipment [IV pole]; weak from surgery)

- Potential alteration in glucose metabolism
  (history of type 2 diabetes)

- Knowledge deficit related to need for help when ambulating
  (unaware of the fall potential and states doesn't need help walking)

- Potential wound infection
  (surgical wound present; history of type 2 diabetes)

- Pain
  (pain still rated at a 7 on a 0 to 10 scale)

- Potential respiratory depression
  (using patient-controlled opioid pain medication)

The problem statements indicate patient care needs based on the evidence collected in Step 1: "Gathering Information."

Step 3 of the Caputi Clinical Judgment Framework requires the nurse to "Determine Actions to Take." Correctly analyzing all the information when *Determining Patient Care Needs* is essential to making good decisions about actions to take.

The second part of this clinical judgment competency of *Determining Patient Care Needs/Healthcare Environment Issues* is *Determining Healthcare Environment Issues*. An example of a healthcare environment issue previously presented in this chapter with the clinical judgment competency of *Recognizing Inconsistencies* is the issue of the nursing assistant stating all the vital signs for 10 patients were taken and recorded in 20 minutes. The nurse suspected a possible inconsistency with that information because the amount of time in which the vital signs were taken and recorded is not consistent with the time expected to complete the task. The nurse must take this information and apply the clinical judgment competency of *Determining Healthcare Environment Issues*. In so doing the nurse determines the healthcare environment issue is: Need for Oversight of Nursing Assistant Related to Technique for Taking and Recording Vital Signs. This issue will be approached using the same clinical judgment framework as applied to patient care needs. The nurse will implement Steps 3, 4, and 5 to work to resolve the issue.

Cognitive Guidance Tool for the Clinical Judgment Competency of "Determining Patient Care Needs/Healthcare Environment Issues"

COGNITIVE GUIDANCE TOOL

The end product of Step 2: "Making Meaning of the Information" is a clear statement of any problem, issue, concern, or care need identified when analyzing the information collected in Step 1: "Getting the Information." As is evident in this chapter, merely gathering information is not enough. The nurse must make meaning of that information concluding with an accurate statement of what needs to be addressed. This process is used when addressing patient care needs as well as issues within the healthcare environment.

This tool guides your use of the clinical judgment competency of *Determining Patient Care Needs/Healthcare Environment Issues*. There are many times you will use this clinical judgment competency in a variety of situations. This tool is just one example. Fill in the information or answer the questions on a piece of paper or use an electronic device as instructed by your faculty.

Determining Patient Care Needs

One reason patients experience adverse outcomes is due to failure to diagnose or identify patient care needs, including changes in the patient condition. Nurses "trend" data over time to determine if changes are occurring.

Complete Table 4.11 with information you gathered from your adult patient and the patient's record. Use that information to compare the current data to the previous 24-hour data.

TABLE 4.11

Comparing Patient Data

Area of Assessment	Normal Findings for THIS Patient	Patient's Current Data	Patient Data 12 Hours Ago	Patient Data 24 Hours Ago
Blood pressure				
Heart rate (beats per minute)				
Respiratory rate (breaths per minute)				
Oxygen saturations (%)				
LOC				
Oriented to person, place, time, and situation				
Temperature				
Intake				
Output				

Add more rows as needed

Analyze the above information using the thinking of the other clinical judgment competencies in Step 2: "Making Meaning of Information" in order to *Determine Patient Care Needs*.

CHAPTER 4 ■ Step 2: Making Meaning of the Information (NCLEX® ~ Analyze Cues) 141

Answer the following questions:

Question
How do the current findings compare with those 12 hours ago and 24 hours ago?

Question
Based on the information, is the patient's condition improving, staying the same, or worsening?

Question
Based on your current level of nursing knowledge, what care needs or issues can you identify?

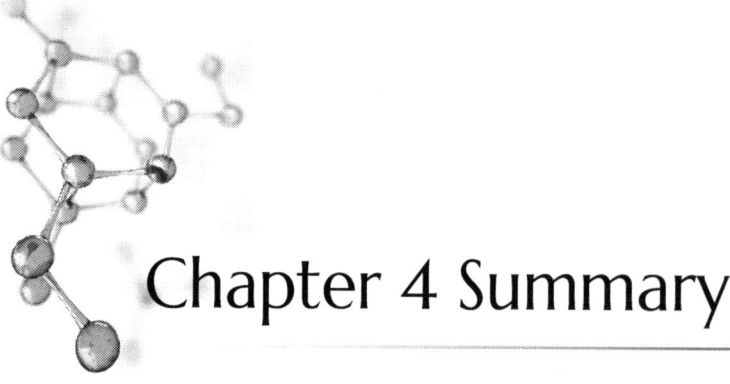

Chapter 4 Summary

This chapter covered...

Step 2 of the Caputi Clinical Judgment Framework:
"MAKING MEANING OF THE INFORMATION"

Presented in this chapter were each of the nine clinical judgment competencies:

1. Clustering related information
2. Identifying assumptions
3. Recognizing inconsistencies
4. Distinguishing relevant from irrelevant information
5. Judging how much ambiguity is acceptable
6. Comparing and contrasting
7. Predicting potential complications
8. Collaborating with healthcare team members
9. Determining patient care needs/healthcare environment issues

Table 4.12 was first presented at the beginning of this chapter. This table demonstrates how the second step of the Caputi Clinical Judgment Framework aligns with the Clinical Judgment Measurement Model of the NCLEX's cognitive process of "Analyze Cues" and the step of the nursing process "Diagnosing."

TABLE 4.12

Alignment of the NCSBN Clinical Judgment Measurement Model, the Caputi Clinical Judgment Framework, and the Steps of the Nursing Process

The Cognitive Processes of the NCSBN Clinical Judgment Measurement Model (Next Generation NCLEX)	Major Steps in the Caputi Clinical Judgment Framework	Steps of the Nursing Process
1. Recognize Cues	Getting the Information	Assessing
2. Analyze Cues	Making Meaning of the Information	Diagnosing
3. Prioritize Hypotheses	Determining Actions to Take	Planning
4. Generate Solutions	Determining Actions to Take	Planning
5. Take Actions	Taking Action	Implementing
6. Evaluate Outcomes	Evaluating Outcomes and Your Thinking	Evaluating

Both the Clinical Judgment Measurement Model of the NCLEX and the nursing process list steps that are general. These steps do not provide the specific thinking (clinical judgment competencies) required with each of these processes. The Caputi Clinical Judgment Framework fills in those missing pieces. These nine clinical judgment competencies form the basis for thinking that will be expected on the NCLEX exam as it measures the candidate's ability to engage in the cognitive process of "Analyze Cues." Success on the NCLEX requires being able to think using these very detailed thinking competencies.

These clinical judgment competencies represent the type of thinking you use when implementing the "Diagnosing" step of the nursing process. To ensure your thinking supports both the "Analyze Cues" cognitive process and the "Diagnosing" step of the nursing process, you must use the detailed thinking of each of these nine clinical judgment competencies.

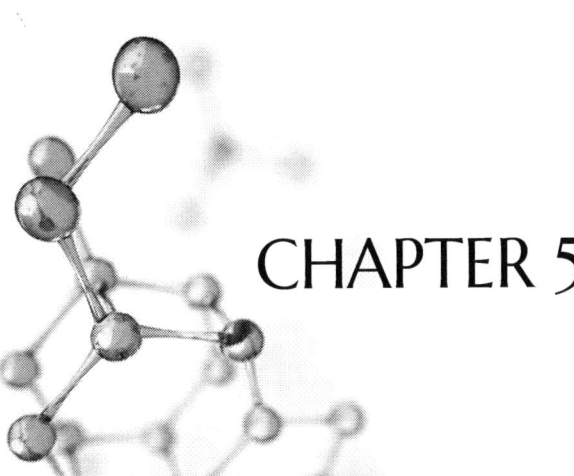

CHAPTER 5

Step 3: Determining Actions to Take
(NCLEX® ~ Prioritize Hypotheses & Generate Solutions)

TABLE 5.1

The Caputi Clinical Judgment Framework: Step 3

Major Steps in the Caputi Clinical Judgment Framework	The Caputi Clinical Judgment Competencies
STEP 1 ~ Getting the Information	• Determining important information to collect • Scanning the environment • Identifying signs and symptoms • Assessing systematically and comprehensively • Ensuring accurate information
STEP 2 ~ Making Meaning of the Information	• Clustering related information • Identifying assumptions • Recognizing inconsistencies • Distinguishing relevant from irrelevant information • Judging how much ambiguity is acceptable • Comparing and contrasting • Predicting potential complications • Collaborating with healthcare team members • Determining patient care needs/healthcare environment issues
STEP 3 ~ Determining Actions to Take	• Selecting interventions • Managing potential complications • Setting priorities
STEP 4 ~ Taking Action	• Determining how to implement the planned interventions • Delegating • Communicating • Teaching others
STEP 5 ~ Evaluating Outcomes and Your Thinking	• Evaluating data • Evaluating and correcting thinking

Chapter Note:

If you are reading this chapter without first reading Chapter 3, please return to the first part of Chapter 3 and read the following sections:

- How the Content is Presented
- Using the Clinical Judgment Competencies

As shown in Table 5.1, this chapter presents the clinical judgment competencies of Step 3: "Determining Actions to Take" of the Caputi Clinical Judgment Framework. This step is all about making decisions about nursing actions to take based on the thinking processes performed in Steps 1 and 2.

Table 5.2 demonstrates how the "Determining Actions to Take" step aligns with the NCSBN's cognitive processes of "Prioritize Hypotheses" and "Generate Solutions" (NCSBN, 2019) and the Planning step of the nursing process. **Remember**, the Caputi Clinical Judgment Framework is the detailed thinking used with the six cognitive processes that are tested on the Next Generation NCLEX and the thinking behind the nursing process. This is demonstrated with Tables 5.2 and 5.3.

TABLE 5.2

Alignment of the NCSBN Clinical Judgment Measurement Model, the Caputi Clinical Judgment Framework, and the Steps of the Nursing Process

The Cognitive Processes of the NCSBN Clinical Judgment Measurement Model (Next Generation NCLEX)	Major Steps in the Caputi Clinical Judgment Framework	Steps of the Nursing Process
1. Recognize Cues	Getting the Information	Assessing
2. Analyze Cues	Making Meaning of the Information	Diagnosing
3. Prioritize Hypotheses	Determining Actions to Take	Planning
4. Generate Solutions	Determining Actions to Take	Planning
5. Take Actions	Taking Action	Implementing
6. Evaluate Outcomes	Evaluating Outcomes and Your Thinking	Evaluating

Table 5.3 lists the specific thinking processes (clinical judgment competencies) that are needed to be skillful at implementing the "Prioritize Hypotheses" and "Generate Solutions" cognitive processes of the NCSBN's Clinical Judgment Measurement Model that is tested on the Next Gen NCLEX. It will be difficult to "Prioritize Hypotheses" and "Generate Solutions" without learning the detailed thinking that supports that type of thinking.

TABLE 5.3

Prioritize Hypotheses and Generate Solutions (Next Gen NCLEX Cognitive Processes) aligned to the Clinical Judgment Competencies of "Determining Actions to Take"

NCSBN's Clinical Judgment Measurement Model Cognitive Processes	Clinical Judgment Competencies in Caputi's "Determining Actions to Take" Step
Generate Solutions	Selecting Interventions Managing Potential Complications
Prioritize Hypotheses	Setting Priorities

The clinical judgment competencies used in Step 1: "Getting the Information" yield information about the individual patient situation or a situation in the healthcare environment. Step 2: "Making Meaning of the Information" requires analysis of the data to make sense of all the data collected. Both those steps prepare you to determine actions to take either for the patient's care or to deal with an issue in the healthcare environment.

In Step 3 "Determining Actions to Take" you must address the patient care needs/healthcare issues to determine what you need to do. Now that the issues, problems, concerns, or needs are identified, you first plan goals—where you want to "go" compared to where you are now. For example, if the patient care need relates to pain, what is the pain level now and what pain level will you plan as a goal after the patient receives the medication and other pain-relieving measures are implemented? Where are you now and where do you want to be? That is the question. In "Making Meaning of the Information" you were able to clearly identify where you are now—in "Determining Actions to Take" you will determine where you want to go (identify expected outcomes) and plan how you will get there.

When developing your plan of care or plan of action you must consider a number of factors. These factors include:

1. ***Legal, ethical, and professional guidelines*** to ensure your plan is acceptable. This means you must have knowledge of these guidelines, which is part of your nursing education.

2. ***Policies and procedures of the healthcare institution*** to provide specific information about how to carry out nursing care and nursing actions in that agency.

3. ***Position descriptions for others with whom you work.*** For example, if you are working with a nursing assistant, you must be aware of the job description for that position.

4. ***The environment in which you are working which will determine resources available to you.*** For example, you may be caring for a patient in a long-term care facility, in an acute care facility, in the patient's home, or in a clinic. Each of these care environments provide ready resources; however, what those resources are differ greatly depending on the environment.

5. ***Individual patient factors.*** When planning goals and selecting interventions you must always consider the patient's history and demographics as part of the patient's situation. History data include other health-related pre-existing conditions and the patient's social support system. Examples of demographic data to consider for the individual patient include age, gender, educational level, culture, ethnicity, and the patient's adherence to cultural and ethnic norms. Other individual factors may include sexual orientation, gender identity, relationship status, religion, spiritual beliefs, and other issues important to the patient and important for the nurse to consider when planning care for the patient.

Consider these factors when developing your plan of care/action:

Legal, ethical, and professional guidelines

Policies and procedures of the healthcare institution

Position descriptions for others with whom you work

The environment in which you are working which will determine resources available to you

Individual patient factors

The above factors are ones you apply when considering the general healthcare environment in which you work. Knowledge of these factors is used as you then consider actions to take for each individual patient to provide patient-centered care that is situation base—based on full knowledge of the patient's situation. Each of these factors related to the general healthcare environment and specific to the individual patient impacts the planning of nursing actions that best address the patient's care needs or the presenting healthcare environment issue.

All these factors related to the general healthcare environment and specific to the individual patient impact the planning of nursing interventions that best address the patient's care needs or the presenting healthcare environment issue.

CHAPTER 5 ■ Step 3: Determining Actions to Take (NCLEX® ~ Prioritize Hypotheses & Generate Solutions)

CLINICAL JUDGMENT COMPETENCIES

SELECTING INTERVENTIONS

STEP 3: Determining Actions to Take

Definition of "Selecting Interventions"

Selecting Interventions means determining what actions to take based on what needs to be accomplished. Therefore, the first task is to identify a goal to be accomplished. Once the goal is established, actions are planned to meet that goal.

selecting interventions ~ determining what actions to take based on what needs to be accomplished

There are many times when there is only one action that can be taken in a situation so the term "selecting" may not involve making a choice but just knowing what specific action to take in a particular situation. For example, if the nurse determines the patient has no pulse and is not breathing and the patient wishes emergency actions to be taken, the nurse would immediately start cardiopulmonary resuscitation (CPR). There is not a list of actions from which to choose. Performing CPR is the only action to take. Conversely, if the patient is found to have no pulse and is not breathing and there is a specific directive by the patient and the primary care provider to not resuscitate (known as a Do Not Resuscitate [DNR] order), the action selected would be to **not** institute CPR.

An important aspect of *Selecting Interventions* is to determine if there are interventions that are inappropriate. In this example, for a patient who has legally indicated the desire to decline CPR, starting CPR would be inappropriate. This extreme example is used to make clear the nurse's responsibility to ensure the appropriateness of the interventions implemented. In most cases, there are several interventions that can be selected, but the nurse must determine which best meet the patient's needs considering the five factors listed at the beginning of this chapter including all factors related to the individual patient situation.

An important aspect of Selecting Interventions is to determine if there are interventions that are inappropriate.

Another aspect of *Selecting Interventions* addresses monitoring the patient based on issues or concerns that are occurring. For example, if the patient's urinary output from the previous 12 hours was low, the nurse will include a nursing action of "monitor urinary output." The nurse will set a parameter. A parameter indicates the uppermost value and the lowermost value for a specific measurement that is acceptable for that patient. Values outside that range would trigger the nurse to take action. For urinary output, the important lowermost value is 30 milliliters of urine per hour. If the patient's urinary output falls below the lower value as set with the parameter, the nurse would take action.

Another example of a parameter is a patient's heart rate. The typical parameter for the heart rate is the normal range of no lower than 60 beats per minute or higher than 100 beats per minute. However, a particular patient's normal range or physical condition may affect the parameter the nurse sets. If a patient's normal heart rate is between 48 and 54, the nurse would set the lower value at 48. This again demonstrates the need for ensuring all patient care decisions consider the individual patient situation.

Example Using "Selecting Interventions" in Everyday Life

Planning to run a marathon takes time. The goal is to complete the marathon. The runner must select interventions to prepare to meet that goal. Interventions might include running a specific distance each day, engaging in strengthening exercises, following a specific diet plan, and ensuring adequate rest. The interventions selected must be appropriate for the goal of completing the marathon.

Thinking Challenge

Provide an example of how you use the clinical judgment competency of *Selecting Interventions* in your everyday life.

Example Using "Selecting Interventions" in Nursing

The nurse is conducting a health history for a female patient. While "Getting the Information" about the patient's diet, the nurse discovered the patient eats foods high in fat and high in sugar. When "Making Meaning of the Information" the nurse determined a patient care need of eating a healthy diet. The nurse and patient together set a goal of eating a diet low in fat (intake of no more than 44 grams per day) and low in sugar (less than 25 grams per day).

The *Selected Interventions* include assisting the patient to develop a plan with food selections that are low in fat and sugar:

- Eliminate animal fats, saturated fats, and fried food
- Eat healthy fats such as those found in salmon and other fish, and avocados
- Eliminate all sweets
- Read all food labels to identify foods high in sugar and eliminate those from the diet

Cognitive Guidance Tool for the Clinical Judgment Competency of "Selecting Interventions"

Planning patient care by identifying goals and *Selecting Interventions* is also known as developing a patient or nursing care plan. The development of that plan of care can be formal in that it is written and maintained as part of the patient's medical record. Or, planning care can be informal. Informal planning happens continuously throughout the time a nurse is with a patient. The nurse immediately identifies many patient needs, intuitively determines a goal that needs to be met, then *Selects Interventions* to immediately implement. For example, a patient may appear to be in an uncomfortable position in the bed and is having difficulty moving himself to a better position. Informally, the nurse identifies the patient's care need of an uncomfortable position but unable to reposition self, establishes the goal of proper positioning, and *Selects Interventions* such as repositioning the patient and using pillows or other devices to help the patient maintain that position.

Selecting Interventions is based on individual patient needs. Interventions are patient-centered and selected to meet the individual patient needs after understanding the total patient situation. *Selecting Interventions* requires situation-based thinking as discussed in Chapter 1.

The following tool guides your use of the clinical judgment competency of *Selecting Interventions*. There are many times you will use this clinical judgment competency in a variety of situations. This tool is just one example. Fill in the information or answer the questions on a piece of paper or use an electronic device as instructed by your faculty.

COGNITIVE GUIDANCE
TOOL

Selecting Interventions is based on individual patient needs. Interventions are patient-centered and selected to meet the individual patient needs after understanding the total patient situation. Selecting Interventions requires situation-based thinking as discussed in Chapter 1.

Selecting Interventions to Address Patient Care Needs

You are familiar this activity because this cognitive guidance tool was introduced in Chapter 4 for the clinical judgment competency of *Determining Patient Care Needs*.

*Complete Table 5.4 with information you gathered
from your patient and the patient's record,
then use the information to Select Interventions.*

TABLE 5.4

Selecting Interventions

Area of Assessment	Patient's Current Data	Patient Data 12 Hours Ago	Patient Data 24 Hours Ago
Blood pressure			
Heart rate (beats per minute)			
Respiratory Rate (breaths per minute)			
Oxygen saturations (%)			
LOC			
Oriented to person, place, time, and situation			
Temperature			
Intake			
Output			
Pain score (0-10)			

*After you complete Table 5.4,
start your thinking by addressing the same questions
you answered in Chapter 4 for this activity.*

*Analyze the information recorded in the three columns
using the thinking of the clinical judgment competencies
in Step 2 to Determine Patient Care Needs.*

Answer the following questions:

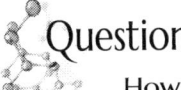
Question
How do the current findings compare with those over the last 24 hours?

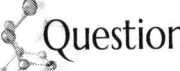
Question
Based on the information, is the patient's condition improving, staying the same, or worsening?

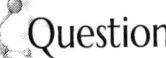
Question
Based on your current level of nursing knowledge, what care needs or issues can you identify?

Now complete Table 5.5. Identify any information indicating a patient need, concern, or problem that must be addressed. Based on your level of nursing knowledge at this time, determine parameters or ranges of acceptable results, then establish a goal and select interventions you will implement to address the identified patient need/concern.

TABLE 5.5

Identifying Patient-Specific Interventions

Patient Care Need/Concern	Parameters for this Patient	Goal	Interventions

Add more rows as needed

STEP 3: Determining Actions to Take

CLINICAL JUDGMENT COMPETENCIES

MANAGING POTENTIAL COMPLICATIONS

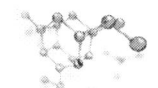

managing potential complications ~

thinking ahead to determine what to do to prevent a complication from happening and what to do should a complication occur in a specific situation

Being prepared for unexpected complications requires clinical forethought because time is often a factor influencing patient outcomes.

Implementing the clinical judgment competencies of Predicting Potential Complications and Managing Potential Complications contributes immensely to keeping your patients safe.

Definition of "Managing Potential Complications"

Managing Potential Complications means thinking ahead to determine what to do to prevent a complication from happening and what to do should a complication occur in a specific situation. That is, what will you do if something goes wrong **and** how will you prevent a potential complication from occurring? Being prepared for unexpected complications requires clinical forethought because time is often a factor influencing patient outcomes. The quicker an unexpected outcome is addressed, the better the chance for achieving a quality outcome. A delayed response to the unexpected outcome can negatively influence patient outcomes. It is always best to prevent a complication from ever happening, rather than dealing with an actual complication. However, should a complication occur, the quicker the complication can be managed (the time factor), the less likely the patient will experience harm or an adverse reaction to the complication.

As discussed in Chapter 1, a major reason to thoroughly learn about clinical judgment is to ensure you are able to deal with unexpected occurrences and to reduce errors in the healthcare setting. One action for meeting this goal was carried out in Step 2 "Making Meaning of the Information" when you engaged in *Predicting Potential Complications*. The clinical judgment competency of *Managing Potential Complications* ensures you have engaged in clinical forethought to be prepared to deal with potential complications you identified. This reduces the risk of unexpected occurrences from happening because you identified them before they occurred. Of course, there is no assurance you will identify every unexpected occurrence, but implementing the clinical judgment competencies of *Predicting Potential Complications* and *Managing Potential Complications* contributes immensely to keeping your patients safe.

Example Using "Managing Potential Complications" in Everyday Life

A common complication in everyday life is a problem with traffic. You are driving to work and signs begin to appear that alert you to construction ahead. Traffic is starting to slow. You look at the GPS which notes slowed then stopped traffic for the next five miles. As you consider this information you predict there is a potential complication related to driving to work because of backed up traffic. You consider the further complications that may result if you do not arrive at your destination on time. The complications are:

- Late for work
- Run out of gas

To manage complications, you begin to consider interventions to implement. These interventions might include:

- Take the next exit which is in one mile; the GPS indicates the traffic on the alternate route is slow but not stopped
- Stay on the route and notify your employer of a likely late arrival
- Locate nearest gas station on the route

Thinking Challenge

Provide an example of how you use the clinical judgment competency of *Managing Potential Complications* in your everyday life.

Example Using "Managing Potential Complications" in Nursing

Some patients in the acute care setting receive opioid analgesics (e. g. codeine, morphine, hydromorphone, fentanyl) to control pain. Some opioids can be administered intravenously using an on-demand system where the patient self-administers the drug by pushing a button to release a dose of the medication. This is called patient-controlled analgesia (PCA). A potential complication of PCA is a decreased respiratory rate. The nurse knows to closely monitor the patient's respiratory rate. However, should the respiratory rate drop too low, perhaps below 12 breaths per minute, the nurse must know how to manage this complication.

Planning what to do prior to the event actually happening is extremely important and is known as clinical forethought. The nurse prepares for *Managing Potential Complications* by using the clinical judgment competency of *Predicting Potential Complications* during the "Making Meaning of the Information" step. In the "Determining Actions to Take" step the nurse addresses how to manage the identified potential complications. Although presented in this book as clearly two different clinical judgment competencies in the clinical judgment process, the nurse automatically carries out these two clinical judgment competencies together.

COGNITIVE GUIDANCE TOOL

Cognitive Guidance Tool for the Clinical Judgment Competency of "Managing Potential Complications"

Two common reasons for adverse (poor) patient outcomes are failure to institute appropriate treatment and inappropriate management of complications (Andel, et al., 2012). Planning ahead to determine appropriate treatment and management of complications can improve patient outcomes.

This tool guides your use of the clinical judgment competency of *Managing Potential Complications*. There are many times you will use this clinical judgment competency in a variety of situations. This tool is just one example. Fill in the information or answer the questions on a piece of paper or use an electronic device as instructed by your faculty.

Managing Potential Complications Once Potential Complications Are Identified

This cognitive guidance tool has two steps. Step 1 will be familiar to you. It is the cognitive guidance tool used in Chapter 4 for the clinical judgment competency of *Predicting Potential Complications*. Once you complete Step 1, complete Step 2 in which you plan ways to prevent complications from occurring then determine what interventions to take if the complications do occur.

STEP 1:
Analyzing Patient Information to Predict Potential Complications

The following are some commonly occurring individual factors the nurse considers that may put a patient at risk for potential complications.

- Is there anything about this patient that leads you to believe there is a possibility the patient might fall?

- Is the patient physically weak and in need of assistance ambulating?

- Is the patient 65 years of age or older and at risk to fall?
- Is the patient cognitively impaired and not able to follow instructions?
- Does the patient have a sensory loss such as poor hearing or vision?
- Is the patient taking medications that cause dizziness or make the patient drowsy?
- Is the patient on complete bedrest?
- Is the patient overweight?
- Does the patient use tobacco products?
- Does the patient have other pre-existing illnesses?

Based on your current level of nursing knowledge, answer the following questions related to your patient.

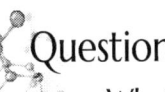
Question
What are you on alert for today with this patient and why?

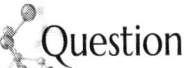
Question
What are the important assessments to make and why?

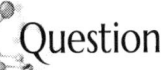
Question
What complications may occur and why?

STEP 2:
Managing Potential Complications

Review the above information for *Predicting Potential Complications*. Use that information to complete the following cognitive guidance tool.

158 Think Like a Nurse: The Caputi Method for Learning Clinical Judgment

*For each of the potential complications you identified,
plan interventions to prevent those complications from occurring.
Complete Table 5.6.*

TABLE 5.6

Planning Interventions to Prevent Potential Complications

Potential complication	Interventions to PREVENT the potential complication from occurring

Add additional rows as needed

*Complete Table 5.7 by explaining what action you will take
should each of the complications actually occur.*

TABLE 5.7

Handling Actual Complications

Potential complication	What you will do should the complication occur

Add additional rows as needed

CLINICAL JUDGMENT COMPETENCIES

SETTING PRIORITIES

STEP 3:

Determining Actions to Take

Definition of "Setting Priorities"

Setting Priorities aligns with the Next Generation NCLEX cognitive process of **Prioritize Hypotheses**. What is a hypothesis? Generally, a hypothesis refers to an explanation of an occurrence, or an explanation of the information collected about a patient determined when using the clinical judgment competencies in the "Making Meaning of the Information" step of clinical judgment. A hypothesis is the nurse's informed explanation about a patient's situation based on known facts and by processing those facts. Therefore, a hypothesis is an explanation resulting from the processing of subjective and objective patient data, or information about some occurrence in the healthcare environment.

Setting Priorities refers to determining which patient issues/concerns are most important and the order in which nursing actions will be taken to address patient care needs or, the order in which to address an issue in the healthcare environment. When faced with a number of choices to make, *Setting Priorities* refers to determining what to do first, second, third, etc. Criteria are used to set priorities. The criteria used may vary according to the situation. In everyday life, the criteria used may align with that used in nursing; such as, what is the most urgent, what will cause harm if not tended to immediately, or what can wait until later. However, in everyday life, criteria may be used that would not be used in nursing. For example, a list of actions might be prioritized according to criteria related to "feelings": What do I feel like doing, washing the dishes or watching TV? *Setting Priorities* in nursing is always patient-centered and based on patient needs.

Setting priorities is a clinical judgment competency constantly used by nurses in all healthcare environments. Prioritizing can be a simple task or a complex task that involves using many other clinical judgment competencies. Nursing examples include:

- Caring for a group of patients and deciding which patients to see first, second, etc.

- For each individual patient, determining which assessments and interventions are most important and must be carried out first.

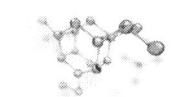

setting priorities ~

determining which patient issues/concerns are most important and the order in which nursing actions will be taken to address patient care needs or issues in the healthcare environment

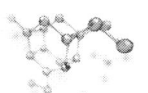

hypothesis ~

an explanation of an occurrence, or of the information collected about a patient determined when using clinical judgment

Prioritizing for a Group of Patients

In some settings, protocols are in place to help a nurse prioritize. For example, triage nurses in the emergency department (ED) typically follow a procedure in which patients presenting with chest pain or other cardiac symptoms take priority. For patients experiencing less urgent issues, ED nurses use their established knowledge base and experience to determine which patients must be seen first based on the individual patient situation.

Prioritizing for an Individual Patient

The NCSBN (https://www.ncsbn.org/13342.htm) lists "Prioritize Hypotheses" as a major cognitive process tested on the Next Generation NCLEX. To prioritize hypotheses, the NCSBN suggests students look at patient care needs and rank them according to guidelines such as urgency, likelihood of complications occurring, and time, that is in what amount of time will the patient experience consequences if the nursing intervention is not implemented. Some of the questions nurses consider when prioritizing nursing interventions for an individual patient include:

1. Which findings require immediate attention or immediate follow-up?
2. Which nursing actions are **not** immediately necessary?
3. What are the consequences if an action is not implemented?
4. What are the top 3 priority nursing actions?
5. Which nursing interventions can be implemented in the amount of time available?
6. In what amount of time will an adverse reaction occur if the necessary nursing interventions are not taken?

The cognitive guidance tool for this clinical judgment competency provides practice with prioritizing nursing interventions for an individual patient.

Example Using "Setting Priorities" in Everyday Life

Setting priorities is a very common clinical judgment competency used in everyday life. You may set and reset priorities many times throughout the day. One example is forgetting to set your alarm and you over-sleep. You eventually wake up, but you wake up a half hour late. You typically need one and a half hours to get ready for work in the morning. Since you are a half hour late, you must now revise your normal routine. Some of the routine tasks may not get done. How do you reset your priorities with the reduced amount of time? On a typical morning after you wake up you:

- Exercise
- Shower
- Dress
- Eat breakfast
- Gather all your materials for work
- Walk the dog

Waking up late, you must now reprioritize this list and perhaps even change the items on the list. In this example, time is a factor that influences how you will prioritize. You ask yourself:

- What tasks must be done?
- What tasks can be left undone?
- What are the consequences if a task is left undone?

You then prioritize what you can do in an hour rather than the typical one and a half hours you need to get ready for work.

Thinking Challenge

Provide an example of how you use the clinical judgment competency of *Setting Priorities* in your everyday life.

Example Using "Setting Priorities" in Nursing

Setting Priorities is a clinical judgment competency constantly used by nurses in all areas of nursing. For example, the nurse is caring for five patients and is working with one nursing assistant. After receiving report from the nurse on the previous shift, the nurse must prioritize what to do. A major force that influences the task of setting priorities is patient safety. To ensure all five patients are safe, the nurse determines the order in which to visit each patient. Information from the shift report guides the nurse's thinking about how to prioritize. Some factors to consider include:

A major force that influences the task of setting priorities is patient safety.

- The stability of each patient's condition: That is, are any of the patient's conditions changing frequently and do these patients need close monitoring?
- Are any patients at risk for injury due to conditions such as confusion or dizziness?
- Are any patients requesting, or are due for, scheduled pain medication?
- Do any patients have time-sensitive medications to be administered immediately such as a cardiac medication or insulin? (Time-sensitive means the medication must be delivered at a specific time or it will have negative results. For example, certain cardiac medications must be taken at specific intervals; some insulins must be given before a meal.)

These are examples of factors nurses consider when determining how to prioritize their work. Every environment is different thus the factors to consider when prioritizing varies depending on the patient population (patients in the ED versus on a general surgical unit), the individual patient situation (unstable versus stable), and the healthcare setting (acute care, long-term care, home environment).

COGNITIVE GUIDANCE TOOL

Cognitive Guidance Tool for the Clinical Judgment Competency of "Setting Priorities"

Setting Priorities is a central focus for safe patient care. For that reason, the NCLEX has always focused on *Setting Priorities* and does so more intently on the Next Generation NCLEX when measuring the candidate's ability to **Prioritize Hypotheses**. This cognitive guidance tool can get you started *Setting Priorities*.

This tool guides your use of the clinical judgment competency of *Setting Priorities*. There are many times you will use this clinical judgment competency in a variety of situations. This tool is just one example. Fill in the information or answer the questions on a piece of paper or use an electronic device as instructed by your faculty.

Setting Priorities in Nursing Care

There are a number of ways nurses set priorities. This tool uses what is known as the ABCD Prioritization Model for planning individual patient care. There is another prioritizing scheme that uses ABCs which refers to airway, breathing, and circulation. Once the ABCs are established for a patient, and the nurse is ready to provide individual patient care, the ABCD Prioritization Model is used to determine priorities related to the selected nursing interventions. You can think of your selected nursing interventions as your "to-do" list. Your "to-do" list includes everything you need to complete for the patient, but what do you do first?

- **A** (those you must absolutely do now; these are the most important)

- **B** (better get to in the first hour; there can be consequences if these tasks are not completed but you need to finish the interventions listed under "A")

- **C** (can wait for a few hours; these interventions must get done, but can be scheduled into your less busy times)

- **D** (can delegate or assign to an unlicensed care provider; if a nursing intervention can be delegated or assigned then you should do so to free up time for nursing interventions in A, B, and C that cannot be assigned to another care provider)

Review your plan of care for the day.
After assessing your patient, use the ABCD Prioritization Model to answer these questions:

Question
What nursing interventions are needed for your patient today?

Question
What interventions do you consider in the A group (absolutely now)? Explain.

Question
What complications may occur if you do not carry out immediately the interventions in the A group?

Question
What interventions do you consider in the B group (better get to in the first hour)? Explain.

Question

What complications may occur if you do not carry out these interventions within the first hour?

Question

What interventions do you consider in the C group (can wait for a few hours)? Explain.

Question

What interventions do you consider in the D group (can delegate or assign to another care provider)? Explain.

NOTE:

*You will learn about delegation in Chapter 6.
Hold on to this question until that time if you do not feel prepared
to suggest interventions that can be delegated or assigned.*

Some Additional Suggestions

To practice *Setting Priorities* throughout your nursing courses, consider the following questions that summarize what was discussed in this chapter:

1. Which findings require immediate attention or immediate follow-up?

2. What is the most urgent? The most urgent or highest priority needs are ones that are life-threatening. Medium priority problems may not threaten life, but may result in physical or emotional harm.

3. For non-urgent patient needs, are there future consequences if the problem is not addressed?

4. What will cause harm if not tended to immediately?

5. In what amount of time will an adverse reaction occur if the necessary nursing interventions are not taken?

6. Which patients are at risk for injury?

7. What can wait until later?

8. Which nursing actions are not immediately necessary?

9. What are the consequences of an action not implemented?

10. What are the top three priority nursing actions you should perform for this patient?

11. Considering the amount of time available, what nursing interventions must be implemented in the time you have available? Are any patients in need of care where time is of the essence, that is, harm will come if an action is not taken immediately?

12. Which patient is most stable? Least stable? That is, are any of the patient's conditions changing frequently and do these patients need close monitoring?

13. Do any patients have time-sensitive medications to be administered immediately such as a cardiac medication or insulin?

14. Are any patients requesting, or due for pain medication?

Keep this list of questions in your pocket as you care for patients in the clinical setting. Pull out the list as a reminder to keep you focused and mindful when *Setting Priorities* that result in safe patient care.

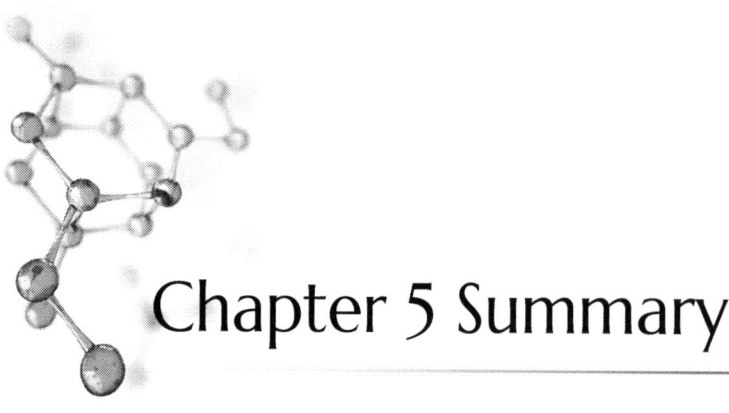

Chapter 5 Summary

This chapter covered...

Step 3 of the Caputi Clinical Judgment Framework:
"DETERMINING ACTIONS TO TAKE"

Presented in this chapter were each of the three clinical judgment competencies:

1. Selecting interventions

2. Managing potential complications

3. Setting priorities

Table 5.8 was first presented at the beginning of this chapter. This table demonstrates how the third step of the Caputi Clinical Judgment Framework aligns with the Clinical Judgment Measurement Model of the NCLEX's cognitive processes of "Prioritize Hypotheses" and "Generate Solutions" and the step of the nursing process "Planning."

TABLE 5.8

Alignment of the NCSBN Clinical Judgment Measurement Model, the Caputi Clinical Judgment Framework, and the Steps of the Nursing Process

The Cognitive Processes of the NCSBN Clinical Judgment Measurement Model (Next Generation NCLEX)	Major Steps in the Caputi Clinical Judgment Framework	Steps of the Nursing Process
1. Recognize Cues	Getting the Information	Assessing
2. Analyze Cues	Making Meaning of the Information	Diagnosing
3. Prioritize Hypotheses	Determining Actions to Take	Planning
4. Generate Solutions	Determining Actions to Take	Planning
5. Take Actions	Taking Action	Implementing
6. Evaluate Outcomes	Evaluating Outcomes and Your Thinking	Evaluating

Both the Clinical Judgment Measurement Model of the NCLEX and the nursing process list steps that are general. These steps do not provide the specific thinking (clinical judgment competencies) required with each of these processes. The Caputi Clinical Judgment Framework fills in those missing pieces. These three clinical judgment competencies form the basis for thinking that will be expected on the NCLEX exam as it measures the candidate's ability to engage in the cognitive processes of "Prioritize Hypotheses" and "Generate Solutions." Success on the NCLEX requires being able to think using these very detailed thinking competencies.

These clinical judgment competencies represent the type of thinking you use when implementing the "Planning" step of the nursing process. To ensure your thinking supports both cognitive processes of the Next Generation NCLEX and the nursing process, you must use the detailed thinking of each of these three clinical judgment competencies.

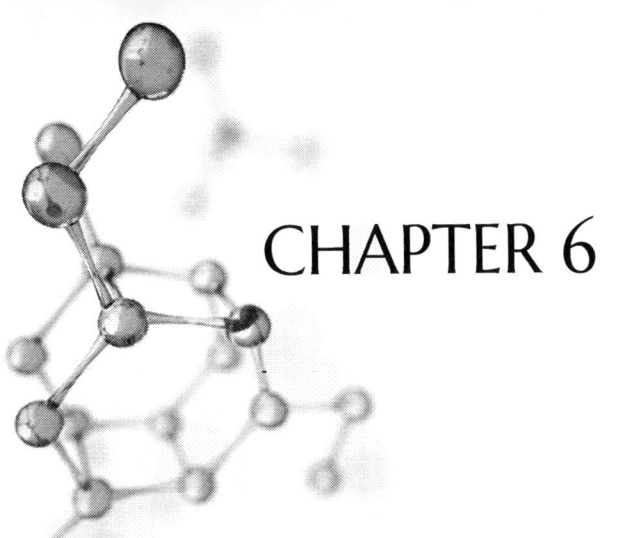

CHAPTER 6

Step 4: Taking Action
(NCLEX®~Take Actions)

TABLE 6.1

The Caputi Clinical Judgment Framework: Step 4

Major Steps in the Caputi Clinical Judgment Framework	The Caputi Clinical Judgment Competencies
STEP 1 ~ Getting the Information	• Determining important information to collect • Scanning the environment • Identifying signs and symptoms • Assessing systematically and comprehensively • Ensuring accurate information
STEP 2 ~ Making Meaning of the Information	• Clustering related information • Identifying assumptions • Recognizing inconsistencies • Distinguishing relevant from irrelevant information • Judging how much ambiguity is acceptable • Comparing and contrasting • Predicting potential complications • Collaborating with healthcare team members • Determining patient care needs/healthcare environment issues
STEP 3 ~ Determining Actions to Take	• Selecting interventions • Managing potential complications • Setting priorities
STEP 4 ~ Taking Action	• Determining how to implement the planned interventions • Delegating • Communicating • Teaching others
STEP 5 ~ Evaluating Outcomes and Your Thinking	• Evaluating data • Evaluating and correcting thinking

Chapter Note:

If you are reading this chapter without first reading Chapter 3, please return to the first part of Chapter 3 and read the following sections:

- How the Content is Presented
- Using the Clinical Judgment Competencies

As shown in Table 6.1, this chapter presents the clinical judgment competencies of Step 4: "Taking Action" of the Caputi Clinical Judgment Framework. This step is all about implementing the actions planned in Step 3: "Determining Actions to Take."

Table 6.2 demonstrates how the "Taking Action" step aligns with the NCSBN's cognitive process of "Take Actions" (NCSBN, 2019) and the Implementing step of the nursing process. **Remember**, the Caputi Clinical Judgment Framework is the detailed thinking used with the six cognitive processes that are tested on the Next Generation NCLEX and the thinking behind the nursing process. This is demonstrated with Tables 6.2 and 6.3.

TABLE 6.2

Alignment of the NCSBN Clinical Judgment Measurement Model, the Caputi Clinical Judgment Framework, and the Steps of the Nursing Process

The Cognitive Processes of the NCSBN Clinical Judgment Measurement Model (Next Generation NCLEX)	Major Steps in the Caputi Clinical Judgment Framework	Steps of the Nursing Process
1. Recognize Cues	Getting the Information	Assessing
2. Analyze Cues	Making Meaning of the Information	Diagnosing
3. Prioritize Hypotheses	Determining Actions to Take	Planning
4. Generate Solutions	Determining Actions to Take	Planning
5. Take Actions	Taking Action	Implementing
6. Evaluate Outcomes	Evaluating Outcomes and Your Thinking	Evaluating

Table 6.3 lists the specific thinking processes (clinical judgment competencies) that are needed to be skillful at implementing the "Take Actions" cognitive process of the NCSBN's Clinical Judgment Measurement Model. It will be difficult to "Take Actions" without learning the detailed thinking that supports this type of thinking.

TABLE 6.3

Take Actions (Next Gen NCLEX Cognitive Process) aligned to the Clinical Judgment Competencies of Step 4: Taking Action

NCSBN's Clinical Judgment Measurement Model Cognitive Process	Clinical Judgment Competencies in Caputi's "Taking Action" Step
Take Actions	Determining How to Implement the Planned Interventions
	Delegating
	Communicating
	Teaching Others

The clinical judgment competencies used in the Step 1: "Getting the Information" yield information about the individual patient situation or a situation in the healthcare environment. Step 2: "Making Meaning of the Information" requires analysis of the data to make sense of all the data collected. Step 3: "Determining Actions to Take" results in stated goals, selecting nursing actions to implement, and prioritizing the nursing actions.

All three steps prepare you for "Taking Action" when caring for the patient or alleviating issues within the healthcare environment. To prepare for "Taking Action," the nurse must determine how to implement the individualized interventions planned. That is, what might need to be changed about a standard, textbook procedure such as inserting a urinary catheter to address the specific patient's needs. This thinking is addressed with the clinical judgment competency of *Determining How to Implement the Planned Interventions*. Other clinical judgment competencies used in this step are *Delegating* (to determine if the intervention can be delegated to another team member), *Communicating* (always an important competency), and *Teaching Others*. *Teaching Others* refers to teaching not only the patient, but to teaching other members of the healthcare team as needed.

The intended result of implementing the "Taking Action" step is to implement the planned actions for the purpose of providing safe patient care. The objective is to realize the goals established. The overall goal may be for the patient to improve with no adverse events occurring, or the overall goal is to assist the patient to experience a peaceful death. In the case of "Taking Action" about a healthcare environment issue, the goal is for the issue to be resolved with evidence the healthcare environment is a safe place for quality patient care.

CLINICAL JUDGMENT COMPETENCIES

DETERMINING HOW TO IMPLEMENT THE PLANNED INTERVENTIONS

STEP 4: Taking Action

Definition of "Determining How to Implement the Planned Interventions"

Step 3: "Determining Actions to Take" provided a plan of action. In Step 4: "Taking Action," actions are taken to implement the plan. The clinical judgment competency of *Determining How to Implement the Planned Interventions* is used to determine exactly how each action will be implemented within the individual patient situation. Many of the planned interventions may have established procedures to follow. The established procedures are used in a majority of cases; however, there are times when the established procedure may have to be adapted to a particular patient situation. Using situation-based thinking, as explained in Chapters 1 and 2, the nurse determines aspects of the situation that influence how the planned interventions are carried out.

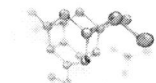

determining how to implement the planned interventions ~

used to determine exactly how each action will be implemented within the individual patient situation

Example Using "Determining How to Implement the Planned Interventions" in Everyday Life

There are many times in everyday life when an action is modified to fit the situation. For example, the instructions for baking a cake on a cake mix box provide information for baking at lower altitudes. The box also provides changes that need to be made when baking at higher altitudes. While *Determining How to Implement the Planned Interventions* the baker must determine the altitude, or height above sea level, of the place where the cake is being baked, then adapt the instructions as noted for baking at higher altitudes.

Another example of using *Determining How to Implement the Planned Interventions* is when a couple are preparing to take their one mile after-dinner walk. The one mile walk is the planned intervention. *Determining How to Implement the Planned Intervention* might involve choosing which route to take based on situational factors such as wanting a variation of scenery, or encountering an obstruction on a previously used route.

Thinking Challenge

Provide an example of how you use the clinical judgment competency of *Determining How to Implement the Planned Interventions* in your everyday life.

Example Using "Determining How to Implement the Planned Interventions" in Nursing

In Step 3 "Determining Actions to Take" the nurse used the clinical judgment competency of *Setting Priorities*. The actions deemed as priority actions are considered first when *Determining How to Implement the Planned Interventions*. If there are several priority actions, the nurse must consider the situation as it now presents to determine which of the priority actions to take first, second, third, and so forth.

During the early terms of a nursing program, students typically learn to perform many nursing skills such as administering an intramuscular injection, inserting a urinary catheter, changing a dressing, and many others. The nursing skills are typically taught using a specific procedure and a list of steps with rationales. The procedure represents the basic information for performing the nursing skill. However, many times the basic information must be changed depending on the individual patient situation. Patient-centered nursing care requires the nurse to adapt, or change, the steps of a nursing skill to address the individual patient situation. Ensuring safety is a major responsibility when making adaptations using the clinical judgment competency of *Determining How to Implement the Planned Interventions*.

There are some steps of a nursing procedure that can never be changed, such as identifying the patient or maintaining sterile technique during a sterile procedure. However, other steps may be safely changed. For example, performing a dressing change includes the step of explaining the procedure to the patient. However, if the patient is an infant or an elderly patient with severe dementia, teaching the patient about the dressing change may not be done, or greatly modified.

> *Patient-centered nursing care requires the nurse to adapt, or change, the steps of a nursing skill to address the individual patient situation.*

> *Ensuring safety is a major responsibility when making adaptations using the clinical judgment competency of Determining How to Implement the Planned Interventions.*

The patient's history that includes pre-existing conditions is also considered when *Determining How to Implement the Planned Interventions*. If the nurse is performing a nursing skill that requires the patient to lie flat, but the patient has a history of a respiratory illness that requires the head of the bed to be elevated at all times, implementation of that nursing skill will be adapted to meet the patient's need to breathe to maintain satisfactory oxygen levels.

It is acceptable to revise the standard textbook procedure for a nursing skill, but only with rationale for the revision. Considerations to make prior to modifying a procedure include:

1. Will the change result in a threat to patient safety—such as not maintaining sterile technique? If so, the change cannot be made.

2. Is the change needed to accommodate a specific patient situation? Can the change be made without putting the patient's safety at risk? Is the change one that needs to be made to achieve quality patient care? If so, it is necessary to make the needed change. It does not help to perform a procedure as written if it does not address the specific, individual patient's needs or puts the patient at risk. Making these changes is part of providing patient-centered care.

Cognitive Guidance Tool for the Clinical Judgment Competency of "Determining How to Implement the Planned Interventions"

COGNITIVE GUIDANCE TOOL

As discussed, textbook procedures provide a suggested way to implement a nursing skill. However, every patient situation needs to be individually considered through a patient-centered, situation-based lens. In so doing, the nurse must *Determine How to Implement the Planned Intervention* in a way that best meets the needs of the patient.

This tool guides your use of the clinical judgment competency of *Determining How to Implement the Planned Interventions*. There are many times you will use this clinical judgment competency in a variety of situations. This tool is just one example. Fill in the information or answer the questions on a piece of paper or on an electronic device as instructed by your faculty.

Adapting a Nursing Skill for the Individual Patient Situation

You are caring for a patient in the clinical setting. Choose a nursing skill you have learned. Although this patient does not have an order for that nursing skill, think about how you might carry out that skill should an order be written.

Complete Table 6.4 by writing in the steps of the nursing skill. Then consider all factors related to your patient's situation and complete the other two columns.

TABLE 6.4

Determining How to Implement a Nursing Skill

Insert Name of Nursing Skill In the rows below insert the steps of the nursing skill.	Can this step in the nursing skill be changed for the individual patient situation? If so, what about the patient's situation requires a change be made to the skill and how will you change it?	Can this step in the nursing skill NOT be changed? Why?

Add additional rows as needed

CLINICAL JUDGMENT COMPETENCIES

DELEGATING

Definition of "Delegating"

Step 4: "Taking Action" of the Caputi Clinical Judgment Framework requires the nurse to determine many factors related to implementing nursing interventions. One factor to consider is "who" will carry out the intervention. *Delegating* addresses this factor. *Delegating* means transferring the responsibility for performing a task to an individual who has been deemed competent to perform that task.

The act of delegating involves many components. The delegator first must ensure the task is something that can be delegated. For example, an adult cannot delegate the task of driving to the store to a teenager who does not yet have a driver's license. Following are some basic, guiding rules about *Delegating* (NCSBN & ANA, 2019):

1. The person to whom the task is delegated must have knowledge about and be able to competently perform the task at hand.

2. The person who is delegating the task must be assured the person is capable of performing the task.

3. The person delegating the task must clearly communicate what is being delegated.

4. The person delegating must ensure appropriate supervision of the task as needed.

5. The person delegating the task must evaluate the results of performance of the task.

6. No task can always be delegated.

Clinical judgment must be used to determine if a task should be delegated. Circumstances about a particular situation can result in not delegating a task which might otherwise be delegated. A task may be delegated to a particular person under certain circumstances, but that same task may not be delegated to that same person under different circumstances. To return to the driving example, an adult may delegate to a newly licensed 16-year-old driver to drive alone to the store five blocks away. However, the task of driving alone in heavy

STEP 4:

Taking Action

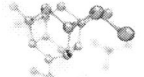

delegating ~
transferring the responsibility for performing a task to an individual who has been deemed competent to perform that task

No task can always be delegated.

traffic on a busy expressway would not be delegated to the same driver. Although the task of driving legally can be delegated to the newly licensed driver, the adult may make a final decision about delegating a specific driving task depending on factors that affect that situation. Driving in heavy traffic adds complexity to the task. Delegating a particular task (in this case driving) is not an absolute but is relative depending on the circumstances of the situation.

Delegating in everyday life requires the same delegation skills that are used in nursing. Delegating requires nurses to engage in assessing, planning, assigning, supervising, and evaluating. Each of these roles requires a high degree of thinking and decision making. When engaging in delegation activities, nurses are accountable for accurately and responsibility carrying out the delegation process in all patient care situations. Prior to delegating a task, the nurse must be familiar with the skill level of the person to whom the task is to be delegated. The nurse must be well informed about the job description of the person to whom the task is delegated and be familiar with the scope of practice as written in the state nurse practice act. Once the delegated task is finished, the nurse must collect data to determine whether the task was performed correctly and the desired outcome was achieved.

Compare these necessary *Delegating* components in nursing to *Delegating* in everyday life. In the case of the young driver, the person delegating the task of driving to the store would carry out the same steps:

1. Accurately and responsibly delegate the task of driving to the store
2. Ensuring the skill level of the person who will perform the driving task
3. Being knowledge about the laws related to driving a motor vehicle
4. Upon completion of the task, collecting data to ensure the task was correctly performed— safe return from the store with the items
5. Holding oneself accountable for delegating the task

The same process used to delegate in everyday life is used when *Delegating* in the form of clinical judgment in nursing. This further demonstrates that you already know how to think like a nurse, it is a matter of being aware of that thinking, then apply that thinking to nursing. That is what this textbook is all about—expanding your thinking processes to nursing in the form of clinical judgment.

> *Delegating requires nurses to engage in assessing, planning, assigning, supervising, and evaluating.*
>
> *Each of these roles requires a high degree of thinking and decision making.*

Example Using "Delegating" in Everyday Life

A family is a group of people. Within that group each family member has a role which often includes responsibilities. For example, Dad may have the responsibility of grocery shopping, Mom may have the responsibility of preparing meals, and the children all have chores or tasks they must perform. If someone in the family is unable to perform their designated task, someone else is asked to do so. *Delegating* is the act of assigning that task to another person. For example, Mom is unable to prepare the meal on Monday evening. The task is delegated to their 15-year-old daughter. However, prior to assigning to the daughter the task of cooking the meal, the mother uses the delegation process. This process includes deciding who is best prepared to perform the task, if that person has the skill level to make the planned meal, and if the person is available to perform that task. Once these decisions are made, the task can be safely delegated. However, thinking ahead about what can go wrong, the mom ensured the dad is home to help should a problem occur.

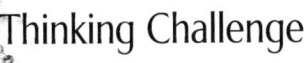

Thinking Challenge

Provide an example of how you use the clinical judgment competency of *Delegating* in your everyday life.

Example Using "Delegating" in Nursing

Delegating is a skill commonly performed by nurses. It is an extremely important responsibility and requires a firm knowledge base. There are important elements to consider, one of which is the state nurse practice act. The nurse practice act in many states indicates which nurses (RNs or LPN/LVNs) are able to delegate nursing tasks to another level of nursing personnel.

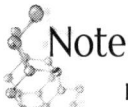

Note:

In some states the LPN/VN cannot **delegate**, rather they **make assignments**. The same guidelines for delegating apply for making assignments. Another element is the agency's job descriptions. The job description for each of the roles: RN, LPN/VN, nursing assistant, and other unlicensed assistive personnel indicates that position's responsibilities and what tasks each is permitted to perform. These are important factors to consider when *Delegating* a nursing task.

The Registered Nurse is assigned six patients. The nursing team consists of the Registered Nurse, a Practical Nurse, and a nursing assistant. The Registered Nurse delegates to the LPN the task of administering oral medication to two of the patients. The Registered Nurse asks the nursing assistant to take and record the vital signs, to ambulate two of the patients, and to feed two of the patients. The Registered Nurse can delegate these tasks because both the LPN and the nursing assistant are competent in performing those tasks, the tasks are included in their job descriptions, and the LPN can administer medications as per the state nurse practice act.

COGNITIVE GUIDANCE

TOOL

Cognitive Guidance Tool for the Clinical Judgment Competency of "Delegating"

As you learn about nursing you will study the process used to guide the nurse when *Delegating*. A critical component of that process is knowing what task can be delegated. Registered Nurses delegate nursing tasks to an LPN/VN or to an unlicensed assistive person such as a Certified Nursing Assistant (CNA). The LPN/VN can also delegate tasks in many states; however, in some states the LPN/VN makes assignments rather than delegates. As discussed, two important documents that provide the basis about who can delegate and to whom to delegate are the nurse practice act for your state and the agency's job descriptions for RN, LPN/VN, and unlicensed assistive personnel.

This tool guides your use of the clinical judgment competency of *Delegating*. There are many times you will use this clinical judgment competency in a variety of situations. This tool is just one example. Fill in the information or answer the questions on a piece of paper or use an electronic device as instructed by your faculty.

To complete this activity, you will need a copy of your state's nurse practice act that discusses scope of practice of the RN and the LPN/VN and the agency's job descriptions. You will use the information in these documents for your "because" explanations in the second and third columns.

Delegating Care to an LPN/VN or CNA

Consider the nursing interventions for your patient today.

In Table 6.5 list at least five nursing interventions, then complete the other two columns.

TABLE 6.5

Delegating Nursing Tasks

Nursing Intervention	I can delegate this intervention to an LPN/VN because....	I can delegate this intervention to a CNA because....

Add additional rows as needed

STEP 4: CLINICAL JUDGMENT COMPETENCIES

Taking Action

COMMUNICATING

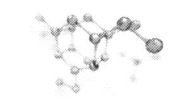

communicating ~

sharing or exchanging thoughts, feelings, or information with others, accomplished through writing, speaking, or facial expressions/ body movements

It is difficult to carry out effective clinical judgment when communication is breaking down.

Definition of "Communicating"

Communicating refers to sharing or exchanging thoughts, feelings, or information with others. *Communicating* is accomplished through writing, speaking, or facial expressions/body movements. Communication involves two people, the sender of the message and the receiver of the message.

Communicating effectively is a highly complex process. Many factors influence communication. Some of these factors include environment, territoriality, values, personal space, attitudes, and time. The nurse must be aware of these and other factors and not let them block effective communication. It is difficult to carry out effective clinical judgment when communication is breaking down.

The principles of therapeutic communication used when interacting with patients, as well as guidelines for positive interpersonal communication when interacting with other healthcare team members, are part of the knowledge base necessary for using the clinical judgment competency of *Communicating* and are essential for safe clinical practice.

Example Using "Communicating" in Everyday Life

People are very social beings and readily communicate with others. Communication is primarily verbal as a child with written and electronic communications included as the person grows and matures. Communicating clearly is often a difficult skill to master. Clear communication with a toddler and child requires different skills than clear communication with an adult.

There are also various types of communication depending on relationships such as social and professional communication. When *Communicating* socially in everyday life, the communication is informal. When everyday life requires *Communicating* with a professional such as lawyer or accountant, the communication is more direct, goal focused, and formal.

Much communication in everyday life is focused on meeting a specific goal such as registering a complaint with a company or inviting others to a party. Any type of communication requires focus and clarity for the communication to be effective. Focus and clarity are communication skills used in everyday life that are valued and applied in nursing. Focusing is part of mindfulness which supports resiliency as discussed in Chapter 1.

Thinking Challenge

Provide an example of how you use the clinical judgment competency of *Communicating* in your everyday life.

Example Using "Communicating" in Nursing

Nurses engage in constant communication throughout their daily practice. They communicate with patients, families, other nursing staff, and other healthcare team members. Communicating in nursing is different from communicating in a social setting. When interacting with patients, family members, and others in the patient's support system, nurses use therapeutic communication techniques and avoid communication techniques that are not therapeutic. Therapeutic communication involves the use of various communication techniques to better understand the patient's needs, concerns, and feelings while helping the patient explore their needs (Burton et al., 2019). Therapeutic communication avoids phrases or words that act as barriers. Examples of a therapeutic communication techniques are: "What can I do to help you this morning?" or "Tell me about how you plan to care for your wound when you go home." Examples of barriers to communication with patients are: "Don't worry, you have the best surgeon in the hospital" or "It's not so bad, other patients are worse off than you." A basic foundations of nursing course will have many examples of therapeutic communication techniques you will use.

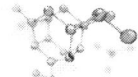

therapeutic communication ~

using various communication techniques to better understand a patient's needs, concerns, and feelings while helping the patient explore their needs.

Communication has a goal and purpose. Nurses focus their communication on the **goal of providing quality patient care for the purpose of improving patient outcomes**. In so doing nurses must be very skilled in providing clear, complete communication.

The term **focus** is very important when *Communicating* with a patient. Nurses must be sure not to allow their minds to wander while the patient is speaking. Refer to the discussion on Mindfulness in Chapter 1 under the topic of becoming resilient. When talking with patients, nurses must clear their minds of other concerns and focus on what the patient is saying. Patients

Nurses focus their communication on the goal of providing quality patient care for the purpose of improving patient outcomes.

soon get the message that what they are saying is not important to the nurse if the nurse's attention is focused on inputting information into the computer or adjusting an IV flow rate during the conversation. Focusing is part of mindfulness which supports resiliency.

Poor communication among healthcare providers is identified as an issue which can result in poor patient outcomes. To ensure communication among all professionals is clear and concise, but complete, most healthcare agencies use a system such as the ISBAR system. The ISBAR mnemonic stands for Identify, Situation, Background, Assessment, and Recommendation(s). Using ISBAR for communicating important information in environments that pose a high risk for error when communication is poor, supports a culture of patient safety.

Completing the ISBAR tool is not a fill-in-the-blanks task. To ensure accurate, complete information is included on the ISBAR form, the nurse must use clinical judgment competencies to think through and select information to include in each of the five parts of the ISBAR tool. Using clinical judgment competencies as you determine what to put on the ISBAR increases the quality of your communication with other healthcare team members.

COGNITIVE GUIDANCE TOOL

Cognitive Guidance Tool for the Clinical Judgment Competency of "Communicating"

This tool guides your use of the clinical judgment competency of *Communicating*. There are many times you will use this clinical judgment competency in a variety of situations. This tool is just one example. Fill in the information or answer the questions on a piece of paper or on an electronic device as instructed by your faculty.

Using Therapeutic Communication

The purpose of this activity is to provide practice using therapeutic communication techniques when *Communicating* with patients, their families, and others in the patient's support system. You will need a list of the therapeutic communication techniques you learned in a nursing course such as fundamentals of nursing. Take the list of therapeutic communication skills to the clinical setting.

After interacting with a patient, leave the room and immediately complete Table 6.6.

TABLE 6.6

Using Therapeutic Communication

Therapeutic communication techniques used with patient	Actual dialogue with patient you had demonstrating the therapeutic technique used	Was the communication effective? Explain.	Was the communication ineffective? Explain.	Ways you can improve your use of the therapeutic communication techniques

Add more rows as needed

Answer the following questions:

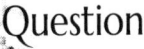

Question

Were you able to identify the therapeutic communication techniques you used?

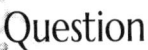

Question

How will you use this experience to improve communication with the patient, their families, and others in their support system?

STEP 4: CLINICAL JUDGMENT COMPETENCIES

Taking Action

TEACHING OTHERS

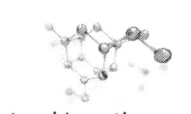

teaching others ~ empowering others with knowledge

Definition of "Teaching Others"

In all aspects of life, teaching empowers others. This is true in nursing; nurses empower patients through teaching.

Teaching Others can occur informally any time a nurse interacts with a patient or when explaining new equipment to a nursing colleague. Teaching is also formal. One example of formalized teaching is discharge teaching, which typically addresses specific areas of care for the patient in preparation for discharge from a healthcare facility. These areas of teaching can include medications, diet, activity restrictions, and follow-up visits. Another example of formalized teaching is diabetic teaching for patients diagnosed with Diabetes Mellitus. This type of formal teaching often involves written guidelines with a checklist to ensure all areas are covered.

Formalized teaching related to *Teaching Others* also includes staff in-service education and training sessions that nurses attend at their place of employment. These sessions are often taught by nurses. In-service offerings may be confined to a unit, or they may be conducted agency-wide when new policies are established that affect many employees. Nurses often lead these teaching sessions.

Clinical judgment is used when carrying out the clinical judgment competency of *Teaching Others*. Nurses consider all factors, looking at the complete patient situation (situation-based nursing), to determine what to include in the individualize teaching plan. For example, discharge teaching has a different focus if the patient is discharged home alone, discharged home with a caregiver, or transferred to an extended-care facility.

Nurses also conduct educational sessions for groups of patients with similar educational needs. Teaching is especially important in the current healthcare environment because many errors and mistakes are made as patients transition from one level of health care to another or from one healthcare facility to another. Some of these errors can be avoided with good patient teaching.

Nurses consider all factors, looking at the complete patient situation (situation-based nursing), to determine what to include in the individualize teaching plan.

Example Using "Teaching Others" in Everyday Life

Teaching and learning occur at all stages of life. Formal teaching occurs in the school environment providing role models for how to teach. Informal environments such as within the family unit or clubs and organizations provide other times in life to experience teaching—both as a teacher and as a learner. Common examples of teaching others in everyday life include teaching a group of children how to play a board game or an outdoor sport, teaching tasks to siblings, teaching an adolescent how to drive a vehicle, or training a new employee.

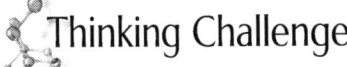

Thinking Challenge

Provide an example of how you use the clinical judgment competency of *Teaching Others* in your everyday life.

Example Using "Teaching Others" in Nursing

Nurses are constantly *Teaching Others*. They teach patients, other healthcare team members, and unlicensed assistive personnel. Some of the teaching is formal such as preoperative teaching for a patient scheduled for surgery. Nurses also teach other nurses about nursing procedures and interventions. Teaching is a major responsibility for nurses.

Teaching Others is often combined with the clinical judgment competency of *Delegating* discussed earlier in this step of the Caputi Clinical Judgment Framework. If the nurse decides to delegate a nursing intervention to another person and the person is unfamiliar with how to proceed, the nurse is responsible for teaching that person how to perform the task and evaluating the learning to ensure the person has learned how to correctly perform the task.

Cognitive Guidance Tool for the Clinical Judgment Competency of "Teaching Others"

COGNITIVE GUIDANCE
TOOL

A major responsibility of the nurse is to teach. Nurses teach patients, their families, other members of the patient's support system, and other healthcare team members. This tool guides your use of the clinical judgment competency of *Teaching Others*. There are many times you will use this clinical judgment competency in a variety of situations. This tool is just one example. Fill in the information or answer the questions on a piece of paper or on an electronic device as instructed by your faculty.

This activity involves teaching patients. Visit your patient and/or the patient's family. Collect information about the patient based on each of the areas listed in Table 6.7.

TABLE 6.7

Planning Patient Teaching

Areas to Assess	Assessment Information for this Patient
Educational Level	
Literacy Level	
Language Spoken	
Social Support	
Financial Resources	
Educational Resources	
Developmental Stage	
Talk with the patient about preferences for learning, such as: "Tell me what is most important to you?" or "What would you like to focus on?"	
Generational Differences Between the Nurse and the Person Being Taught	
Identify Potential or Known Barriers to Learning	

*After completing your assessment,
identify what information is most important
to consider when planning teaching for your patient
by answering the following questions.*

Question

Which are the most important aspects to consider when planning teaching for this patient/family?

Question

Using the information from the assessment table, how will you individualize your teaching?

If this patient is a child, who will you teach in addition to the child such as a parent or guardian?

Question

How will you know whether your teaching was effective?

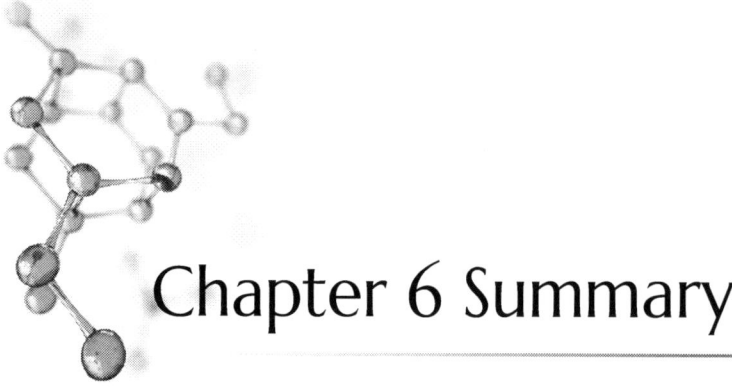

Chapter 6 Summary

This chapter covered...

Step 4 of the Caputi Clinical Judgment Framework:
"TAKING ACTION"

Presented in this chapter were each of the four clinical judgment competencies:

1. Determining how to implement the planned interventions

2. Delegating

3. Communicating

4. Teaching others

Table 6.8 was first presented at the beginning of this chapter. This table demonstrates how the fourth step of the Caputi Clinical Judgment Framework aligns with the Clinical Judgment Measurement Model of the NCLEX's cognitive process of "Take Actions" and the step of the nursing process "Implementing."

TABLE 6.8

Alignment of the NCSBN Clinical Judgment Measurement Model, the Caputi Clinical Judgment Framework, and the Steps of the Nursing Process

The Cognitive Processes of the NCSBN Clinical Judgment Measurement Model (Next Generation NCLEX)	Major Steps in the Caputi Clinical Judgment Framework	Steps of the Nursing Process
1. Recognize Cues	Getting the Information	Assessing
2. Analyze Cues	Making Meaning of the Information	Diagnosing
3. Prioritize Hypotheses	Determining Actions to Take	Planning
4. Generate Solutions	Determining Actions to Take	Planning
5. Take Actions	Taking Action	Implementing
6. Evaluate Outcomes	Evaluating Outcomes and Your Thinking	Evaluating

Both the Clinical Judgment Measurement Model of the NCLEX and the nursing process list steps that are general. These steps do not provide the specific thinking (clinical judgment competencies) required with each of these processes. The Caputi Clinical Judgment Framework fills in those missing pieces. These four clinical judgment competencies form the basis for thinking that will be expected on the NCLEX exam as it measures the candidate's ability to engage in the cognitive process of Take Actions. Success on the NCLEX requires being able to think using these very detailed thinking competencies.

These clinical judgment competencies represent the type of thinking you use when applying the "Implementing" step of the nursing process. To ensure your thinking supports both cognitive processes of the Next Generation NCLEX and the nursing process, you must use the detailed thinking of each of these four clinical judgment competencies.

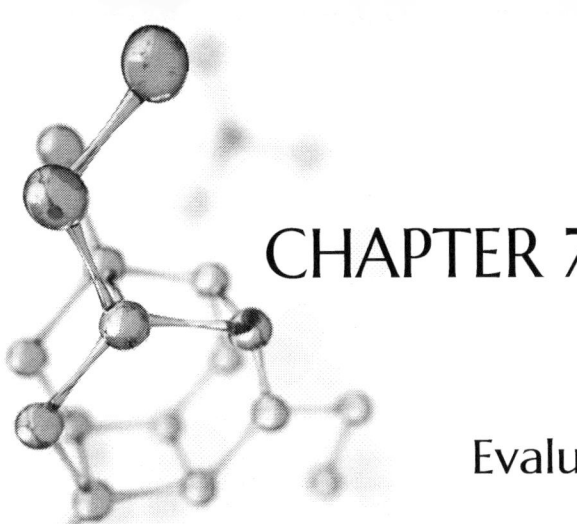

CHAPTER 7

Step 5: Evaluating Outcomes and Your Thinking
(NCLEX®~Evaluate Outcomes)

TABLE 7.1

The Caputi Clinical Judgment Framework: Step 5

Major Steps in the Caputi Clinical Judgment Framework	The Caputi Clinical Judgment Competencies
STEP 1 ~ Getting the Information	• Determining important information to collect • Scanning the environment • Identifying signs and symptoms • Assessing systematically and comprehensively • Ensuring accurate information
STEP 2 ~ Making Meaning of the Information	• Clustering related information • Identifying assumptions • Recognizing inconsistencies • Distinguishing relevant from irrelevant information • Judging how much ambiguity is acceptable • Comparing and contrasting • Predicting potential complications • Collaborating with healthcare team members • Determining patient care needs/healthcare environment issues
STEP 3 ~ Determining Actions to Take	• Selecting interventions • Managing potential complications • Setting priorities
STEP 4 ~ Taking Action	• Determining how to implement the planned interventions • Delegating • Communicating • Teaching others
STEP 5 ~ Evaluating Outcomes and Your Thinking	• Evaluating data • Evaluating and correcting thinking

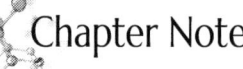 Chapter Note

If you are reading this chapter without first reading Chapter 3, please return to the first part of Chapter 3 and read the following sections:

- How the Content is Presented
- Using the Clinical Judgment Competencies

As shown in Table 7.1, this chapter presents the clinical judgment competencies of Step 5: "Evaluating Outcomes and Your Thinking" of the Caputi Clinical Judgment Framework. This step is all about evaluating the effects of the actions taken in Step 4: Taking Action.

Table 7.2 demonstrates how the "Evaluating Outcomes and Your Thinking" step aligns with the NCSBN's cognitive process of "Evaluate Outcomes" (NCSBN, 2019) and the Evaluating step of the nursing process. **Remember**, the Caputi Clinical Judgment Framework is the detailed thinking used with the six cognitive processes that are tested on the Next Generation NCLEX and the thinking behind the nursing process. This is demonstrated with Tables 7.2 and 7.3.

There is one different aspect of Step 5: "Evaluating Outcomes and Your Thinking" of the Caputi Clinical Judgment Framework from the Evaluate Outcomes step of the NCSBN and the Evaluating step of the nursing process. This difference is the Caputi Framework not only looks at evaluating the effects of actions taken, but also evaluates the thinking used throughout all the steps of clinical judgment framework. To improve thinking, you must constantly reflect on your own thinking to determine whether your thinking led you to the correct actions.

Reflection, as discussed in Chapters 1 and 2, is used for the *Evaluating Your Thinking* clinical judgment competency. Reflecting on your experience is required for the goal of continuously improving your thinking. Merely having an experience isn't enough; you must think back and consider what occurred, what you learned from the experience, and how to use your experience to improve on, or continue using, good clinical judgment. Therefore, reflection is tantamount to learning and growing as a nurse.

> *To improve thinking, you must constantly reflect on your own thinking to determine whether your thinking led you to the correct actions.*

TABLE 7.2

Alignment of the NCSBN Clinical Judgment Measurement Model, the Caputi Clinical Judgment Framework, and the Steps of the Nursing Process

The Cognitive Processes of the NCSBN Clinical Judgment Measurement Model (Next Generation NCLEX)	Major Steps in the Caputi Clinical Judgment Framework	Steps of the Nursing Process
1. Recognize Cues	Getting the Information	Assessing
2. Analyze Cues	Making Meaning of the Information	Diagnosing
3. Prioritize Hypotheses	Determining Actions to Take	Planning
4. Generate Solutions	Determining Actions to Take	Planning
5. Take Actions	Taking Action	Implementing
6. Evaluate Outcomes	Evaluating Outcomes and Your Thinking	Evaluating

Table 7.3 lists the specific clinical judgment competencies (thinking processes) that are needed to be skillful at implementing the "Evaluate Outcomes" cognitive process of the NCSBN's Clinical Judgment Measurement Model. It will be difficult to "Evaluate Outcomes" without learning the detailed thinking that supports evaluating outcomes.

TABLE 7.3

Evaluate Outcomes (Next Gen NCLEX Cognitive Process) Aligned to the Clinical Judgment Competencies of Evaluating Outcomes and Your Thinking

NCSBN's Clinical Judgment Measurement Model Cognitive Process	Clinical Judgment Competencies Taught in Caputi's "Evaluating Outcomes and Your Thinking" Step
Evaluate Outcomes	Evaluating Data Evaluating and Correcting Thinking

> *The intended RESULT of implementing the clinical judgment competency of Evaluating Data is to collect data to determine if the patient's condition is improving, unchanged, or declining.*

> *The intended OUTCOME of the clinical judgment competency of Evaluating and Correcting Thinking is to ensure the entire clinical judgment process the nurse used resulted in good decisions for safe, quality patient care.*

The intended result of implementing the clinical judgment competency of *Evaluating Data* is to collect data to determine if the patient's condition is improving, unchanged, or declining. Close monitoring is critical to identify any indication that the patient's condition is declining so immediate actions can be taken to reverse the declining state.

The nurse also monitors the outcomes of actions taken by others. For example, the nurse is caring for a patient who is two hours post cardiac catheterization. The nurse collects data about the site where the catheter was inserted into the patient's leg. The nurse checks for signs of pain, swelling, and bleeding. The nurse did not perform the cardiac catheterization, but the nurse is responsible to collect evaluation data related to the procedure to ensure the goal of recovering from the procedure is achieved. The nurse is responsible for ensuring no harm comes to the patient related to problems at the insertion site.

The intended outcome of the clinical judgment competency of *Evaluating and Correcting Thinking* is to ensure the entire clinical judgment process the nurse used resulted in good decisions for safe, quality patient care. The goal of this clinical judgment competency is to identify any errors in thinking then develop plans to improve thinking in the future.

CLINICAL JUDGMENT COMPETENCIES

EVALUATING DATA

Definition of "Evaluating Data"

Evaluating Data refers to determining the meaning of the collected evaluation (follow-up) information related to the interventions implemented.

1. Does the follow-up information indicate the issue is resolved or getting better?
2. Does the follow-up information indicate the intervention did not make a difference?
3. Does the follow-up information indicate the condition is worse than the original state?

Chapter 1 listed the reasons for learning clinical judgment. One reason was to **deal with unexpected occurrences and reduce errors in the healthcare setting**. *Evaluating Data* is a clinical judgment competency used to decrease the chance an **unexpected occurrence** will happen. This reason for using clinical judgment is accomplished because the nurse is closely monitoring the patient to determine if interventions are effective or, if not effective, revising the plan of care.

Evaluating Data also works to **reduce errors in the healthcare setting**. Analyzing the collected evaluation data may reveal an error. If an error occurred, the nurse can now intervene to reduce the chance of an unexpected occurrence from happening related to the error. Changes to the plan of care can be made to prevent harm to the patient.

Once actions have been performed, follow-up information (evaluation data) are again collected. Evaluation data are also known as assessment data, but are called evaluation data at this point in the process because the information is used to evaluate the effectiveness of the interventions implemented. Accurate and complete data provide a basis on which to determine further actions to take. The evaluation data and how the data are processed are used to guide continuous, ongoing patient care that may stay the same or change, depending on the evaluation data and whether that data indicate the patient goals have been met.

Evaluating Data yields information to determine if the interventions were effective. Patient data are collected then compared to what was expected when goals were established. When *Selecting Interventions,* the nurse used the process previously explained in Chapter 3 to establish a goal, then *Selected Interventions* intended to achieve that goal. During *Evaluating Data,* the nurse first collects

STEP 5:

Evaluating Outcomes and Your Thinking

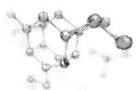

evaluating data ~

determining the meaning of the collected evaluation (follow-up) information related to the interventions implemented

patient data then compares that data to the original data to determine if the outcomes were achieved.

When using the clinical judgment competency of *Evaluating Data* for the purpose of "Evaluating Outcomes," the nurse must be knowledgeable about:

1. **The previous information that indicated the problem, issue, concern.** The nurse must compare the new (evaluation) data to the previously obtained information. Collecting current patient information becomes meaningful when compared to previous information that indicated a patient care need. Nursing interventions were implemented to address that patient need. To determine if the established goal is met, the nurse must be aware of the previous information that indicated there was an issue then compare the evaluation data to that previously identified information.

2. **The patient information (data) that needs to be collected.** The nurse must determine what information to collect; that is, what should be assessed and/or what should be reassessed when collecting evaluation data. That is, what information is directly related to the established goals. Collecting unrelated information will not yield an accurate determination about achievement of the goal. The nurse must ensure the observed and measured outcome information is the information needed to determine achievement of the expected outcomes. The nurse must determine if resources are needed to collect the data; and, if so, ensure those resources are available. For example, the patient shows signs of poor oxygenation. Interventions include increasing the flow rate of the oxygen and positioning the patient for better lung expansion. The nurse will need to measure the patient's oxygen level prior to the interventions then after the interventions. If a pulse oximeter is not available, the nurse must determine how to acquire that needed resource. The pulse oximeter reading represents objective data. The nurse also collects subjective data. In this case, subjective data would include the patient's perspective.

3. **Making meaning of the information when comparing the original information and the evaluation data.** If there are differences, what do the differences mean? For example, if the patient's previous blood pressure was 160/100 and the current blood pressure is 90/50, what does that change indicate? Is the patient's condition improving, unchanged, or deteriorating? A blood pressure of 160/100 is high, so the established goal was

a lower blood pressure. The current blood pressure of 90/50 is certainly lower than 160/100 so it appears the goal has been met. However, is the 90/50 acceptable? Is it too low? The blood pressure of 90/50 is definitely lower than 160/100, but is it within normal limits for this patient? When considering the blood pressure of 90/50 for this particular patient, what does it mean? The nurse must use the clinical judgment competencies of Step 2: "Making Meaning of the Information" to determine if there is now a new patient care need and, if so, work to "Determine Actions to Take." **Note:** An error made in stating the goal for this patient is the lack of a "parameter." A parameter is the acceptable range for the patient's blood pressure. A better stated goal is: Blood pressure between 110/70 and 130/85. With the parameter stated the nurse would make meaning of the 90/50 blood pressure reading and readily determine (1) the blood pressure is lower, (2) there is a new issue to address.

Example Using "Evaluating Data" in Everyday Life

The clinical judgment competency of *Evaluating Data* is used continuously in everyday life, often unconsciously. For example, when making a new recipe for dinner you might evaluate how it tastes and determine what seemed to work best or plan how to improve the recipe for a later time (a little more or a little less of a certain ingredient). As another example, coaches of children's sport teams collect data about how each player performed, determine if additional information is needed, decide how to help each child improve for the next game, or determine a new lineup.

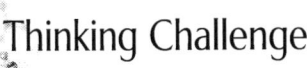
Thinking Challenge

Provide an example of how you use the clinical judgment competency of *Evaluating Data* in your everyday life.

Example Using "Evaluating Data" in Nursing

A simple example of *Evaluating Data* is for a patient experiencing pain. After implementing the first four steps of the Caputi Clinical Judgment Framework, the nurse administered the prescribed opioid analgesia for the patient reporting pain at an 8 on a 0 to 10 scale. The nurse returns to the patient 30 minutes after administering the medication. The patient reports a pain level of 2. The nurse compares the patient's reported pain level of 2 after receiving the medication to the reported pain level of 8 prior to receiving the medication. Additionally, the nurse collects other evaluation data such as the patient's facial expression as a subjective symptom of pain, the patient's report of relief from pain, ease of movement when walking, and manifestations of any adverse effects from the medication such as reports of nausea. When *Evaluating Data* the nurse determines the intervention resulted in improvement of the patient's condition and there are no new concerns related to the intervention.

The nurse administers many medications when caring for patients. The nurse must evaluate the effectiveness of all medications administered to the extent possible. As demonstrated with the previous pain example, evaluating the effectiveness of an analgesic can be fairly straightforward. However, evaluating the effectiveness of other medications might need a little more investigation or might not even be possible. For example, the nurse administers pravastatin to a patient to control blood cholesterol levels for the purpose of preventing a heart attack. The goal of "preventing a heart attack" is actually a long-term goal; therefore, the goal of preventing a heart attack is not a goal the nurse can readily evaluate in the short-term, with the exception of counting each day the patient does not experience a heart attack. For this patient, *Evaluating Data* may focus on monitoring for potential side effects of the drug with the goal of "Early identification of side effects of pravastatin." The nurse may monitor liver enzymes (if ordered) to determine if the patient is experiencing the possible side effect of liver dysfunction or hepatitis.

COGNITIVE GUIDANCE
TOOL

Cognitive Guidance Tool for the Clinical Judgment Competency of "Evaluating Data"

This tool guides your use of the clinical judgment competency of *Evaluating Data*. There are many times you will use this clinical judgment competency in a variety of situations. This tool is just one example. Fill in the information or answer the questions on a piece of paper or on an electronic device as instructed by your faculty.

The *Evaluating Data* clinical judgment competency requires significant information collection and processing. Having an approach to engage in the thinking required is very helpful. The cognitive guidance tool in Table 7.4 helps you organize your thinking as you prepare to engage in the evaluation of patient data you collect. The intent of the tool is to determine what evaluation data to collect, identify the actual information collected, then process that data to determine if the planned interventions were effective.

An alternative approach to using this tool is to consider the data you gather with your initial assessment as evaluation data. You use this data to determine if the nursing interventions previously performed are achieving the established patient goals. It is important that when you start care, you determine if the previous nursing interventions were effective. Why continue to implement the same nursing interventions if those interventions are not meeting the established goals? Nurses evaluate interventions performed by both themselves and other nurses. Because nurses actually do both, perhaps use the tool in both ways as you care for your patient.

TABLE 7.4

Evaluating Data

Previous patient information that indicates a problem, issue, concern	Patient information that needs to be collected to evaluate effectiveness of care	Actual information collected; if not collected, reason why

Add additional rows as needed

Answer the following questions:

Question
Have you collected all necessary data to determine the effectiveness of the interventions?

Question
Do you need to collect additional data?

Question
What specific information indicates the patient's condition is improving?

Question
What specific information indicates the patient's condition is unchanged?

Question
What specific information indicates the patient's condition is declining?

Question
If the condition is unchanged, should the same interventions be used, or should new ones be implemented?

Question
Are there other interventions that would have been more effective than the ones used?

Question
Has a new problem/issue/concern arisen?

The results of *Evaluating Data* provide the basis for determining what further actions are needed.

The answers to the above questions are used to revise the plan of care and determine further interventions available when *Selecting Interventions*.

CLINICAL JUDGMENT COMPETENCIES

EVALUATING AND CORRECTING THINKING

Definition of "Evaluating and Correcting Thinking"

Evaluating and Correcting Thinking refers to determining the quality of the clinical judgment used. When using clinical judgment to resolve a problem, make a decision, or address a patient care need, it is important to evaluate the thinking that occurred. *Evaluating Data*, the previous clinical judgment competency, helps the nurse determine if the actions taken were effective. The *Evaluating and Correcting Thinking* clinical judgment competency is different because it evaluates the thinking used rather than the data collected. This clinical judgment competency requires reflecting on what just happened, how the situation was handled, and what lessons can be learned. The nurse determines if the thinking was accurate or inaccurate. If inaccurate, the nurse considers how the thinking can be improved. Therefore, both *Evaluating Data* and *Evaluating and Correcting Thinking* are critical processes used to provide safe, effective nursing care and to grow as a nurse.

This type of self-evaluation about the thinking processes used promotes professional development, enhances self-confidence, fosters insight into one's own thinking, and promotes better clinical judgment in the future. Implementing the competency of *Evaluating and Correcting Thinking* helps you realize some of the reasons for learning clinical judgment as discussed in Chapter 1: Becoming Resilient, Becoming a Self-Regulated Thinker, and Reducing Errors in the Healthcare Setting.

Reflecting on one's thinking is part of the total clinical judgment process and supports safe patient care. Example questions used to evaluate thinking include:

1. What clinical judgment competencies were used? Were they used effectively?
2. Were the outcomes what was expected? If not, were the outcomes within an acceptable range, or perhaps better than expected?
3. If the outcomes were not acceptable, what might be done differently in the future?
4. How did your thinking impact the people affected, such as the patient, significant others, and other healthcare team members? Was the impact positive or negative?

It is helpful to discuss your thinking (debrief) with your teacher/preceptor. Seek feedback about your use of specific clinical judgment competencies. Ask how the situation could have been handled differently. Use their feedback to improve your thinking.

STEP 5:
Evaluating Outcomes and Your Thinking

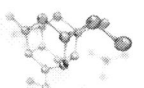

evaluating and correcting thinking ~

determining the quality of the clinical judgment used

Reflecting on one's thinking is part of the total clinical judgment process and supports safe patient care.

Example Using "Evaluating and Correcting Thinking" in Everyday Life

There are many times in everyday life when it is necessary to consider the thinking used to solve a problem. An example might be determining an approach for dealing with a behavioral issue with a child. To deal with the behavior, the parents look at the situation and apply many thinking skills such as:

- *Ensuring accurate information*
- *Clustering related information*
- *Collaborating* with each other or outside counsel
- *Selecting interventions*
- *Determining how to implement the planned interventions*
- *Communicating* with the child about a plan of action

Once the plan is implemented, the parents gather evaluation data about how the child responded to the plan, and if the thinking used led to improved behavior. Perhaps the evaluation data reveal it would have been useful to use the clinical judgment competency of *Teaching Others* by teaching the child about some aspect of the intervention so the child would have been better able to comply.

Although many parents use the thinking competency of *Evaluating and Correcting Thinking* to perfect parenting skills, a formal examination and analysis of their thinking is often missing. *Evaluating and Correcting Thinking* is helpful in everyday life, just as it is in nursing, because you become aware of the thinking used and plan ways to improve.

Thinking Challenge

Provide an example of how you use the clinical judgment competency of *Evaluating and Correcting Thinking* in your everyday life.

Example Using "Evaluating and Correcting Thinking" in Nursing

As nurses evaluate data collected when using the clinical judgment competency of *Evaluating Data*, all expected and unexpected findings are analyzed to determine if the thinking was effective for the individual patient's situation. *Evaluating and Correcting Thinking* is used to determine if the thinking used supports situation-based thinking. That is, did the nurse use the clinical judgment competencies within the individual patient situation—situation-based thinking as discussed in Chapter 1?

Evaluating and Correcting Thinking is used to determine if the thinking used supports situation-based thinking.

If the evaluation data indicate a finding that represents an undesirable outcome, the nurse must review the thinking that occurred and identify if the undesirable outcome was a result of faulty thinking. For example, the nurse notices a patient's call light is on. The nurse is not directly caring for this patient, but enters the patient's room to determine what the patient might need. The patient states he has an urgent need to urinate and requires help to quickly walk to the bathroom. The nurse immediately helps the patient out of bed and begins walking the patient to the bathroom. With the second step the patient falls to the floor and yells, "Don't you know my right side is weak from a stroke I had three years ago!" The nurse immediately takes action to help the patient.

Upon reflecting on this situation, the nurse determined something went wrong with the thinking used to plan how to assist the patient to the bathroom. The nurse immediately identified not using the clinical judgment competency of *Determining Important Information to Collect*. Because the patient was alert and able to talk with the nurse, the nurse could have easily asked the patient if he had any issues with or needed special assistance walking. Once that important information was collected the nurse would have used the clinical judgment competency of *Predicting Potential Complications* (falling) and *Managing Potential Complications* (interventions to prevent a fall). To *Manage the Potential Complication* of falling the nurse might have:

1. Decided there wasn't enough time to walk the patient to the bathroom due to his weakness and offered him a urinal

2. Determined how to support the patient's weak side to safely walk him to the bathroom

This very simple situation analyzing the nurse's thinking, demonstrates the importance of skilled use of the clinical judgment competencies and the ability to apply them as a nurse. The nurse constantly applies the clinical judgment competencies, not just when developing a formal care plan, but throughout all interactions with the patient. Thinking in action is key to safe patient care.

Thinking in action is key to safe patient care.

COGNITIVE GUIDANCE TOOL

Cognitive Guidance Tool for the Clinical Judgment Competency of "Evaluating and Correcting Thinking"

This tool guides your use of the clinical judgment competency of *Evaluating and Correcting Thinking*. There are many times you will use this clinical judgment competency in a variety of situations. This tool is just one example. Fill in the information or answer the questions on a piece of paper or electronic device as instructed by your faculty.

As discussed earlier, after using clinical judgment to identify a problem, issue, or concern, make a decision, and plan and implement patient care, it is important to evaluate the thinking that occurred. *Evaluating Data*, the previous clinical judgment competency in Step 5, helps the nurse determine if the actions were effective. The clinical judgment competency of *Evaluating and Correcting Thinking* is different because it evaluates the **thinking** you used. This clinical judgment competency requires reflecting on what happened, how the situation was handled, and what lessons can be learned to improve your thinking.

Obtaining Feedback on Your Thinking

Complete the activity for the thinking skill of *Evaluating Data* presented in Table 7.4. Once completed, ask your preceptor or faculty for feedback and place that information in the first column of Table 7.5. The best feedback is feedback that addresses specific clinical judgment competencies. Then complete the remaining three columns. Be sure to discuss your use of specific clinical judgment competencies.

TABLE 7.5

Obtaining Feedback on Your Thinking

Feedback from your teacher/preceptor about your thinking	What specific clinical judgment competencies were used correctly and/or incorrectly, or not at all when they should have been used?	Your impression of your thinking	How your impression is the same/different from that of your teacher/preceptor	How you will use the feedback to improve your thinking

Add more rows as needed

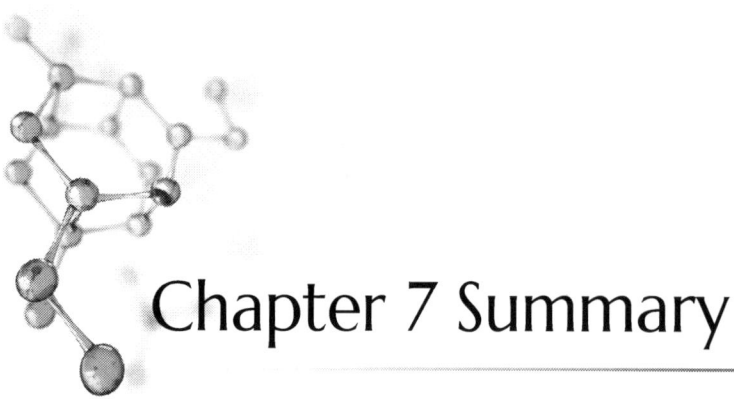

Chapter 7 Summary

This chapter covered...

Step 5 of the Caputi Clinical Judgment Framework:
"EVALUATING OUTCOMES AND YOUR THINKING"

Presented in this chapter were each of the two clinical judgment competencies:

1. Evaluating data

2. Evaluating and correcting thinking

Table 7.6 was first presented at the beginning of this chapter. This table demonstrates how the fifth step of the Caputi Clinical Judgment Framework aligns with the Clinical Judgment Measurement Model of the NCLEX's cognitive process of "Evaluate Outcomes" and the Evaluating step of the nursing process.

TABLE 7.6

Alignment of the NCSBN Clinical Judgment Measurement Model, the Caputi Clinical Judgment Framework, and the Steps of the Nursing Process

The Cognitive Processes of the NCSBN Clinical Judgment Measurement Model (Next Generation NCLEX)	Major Steps in the Caputi Clinical Judgment Framework	Steps of the Nursing Process
1. Recognize Cues	Getting the Information	Assessing
2. Analyze Cues	Making Meaning of the Information	Diagnosing
3. Prioritize Hypotheses	Determining Actions to Take	Planning
4. Generate Solutions	Determining Actions to Take	Planning
5. Take Actions	Taking Action	Implementing
6. Evaluate Outcomes	Evaluating Outcomes and Your Thinking	Evaluating

Both the Clinical Judgment Measurement Model of the NCLEX and the nursing process list steps that are general. These steps do not provide the specific thinking (clinical judgment competencies) required with each of these processes. The Caputi Clinical Judgment Framework fills in those missing pieces. The two clinical judgment competencies discussed in this chapter form the basis for thinking that is expected on the NCLEX exam as it measures the candidate's ability to engage in the NCSBN's cognitive process of Evaluate Outcomes. Success on the NCLEX requires being able to think using these very detailed thinking competencies.

These clinical judgment competencies represent the type of thinking the nurse uses when applying the "Evaluating" step of the nursing process. To ensure your thinking supports the cognitive processes of the Next Generation NCLEX and the nursing process, you must use the detailed thinking of each of these two clinical judgment competencies.

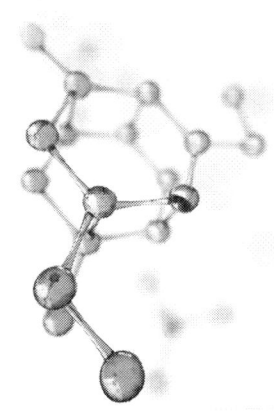
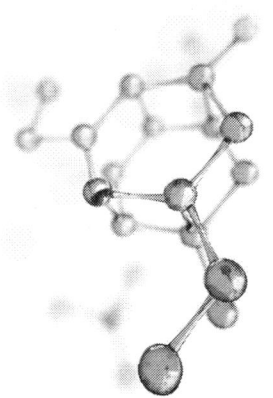

SECTION II

Explaining Your Thinking Using the Caputi Clinical Judgment Framework

(Chapters 8 – 9)

AS DISCUSSED IN SECTION I, your faculty will expect you to explain your thinking and may even ask you to **apply thinking**. Often, the **apply thinking** request does not involve the expectation of an explanation about **how** you were actually thinking, rather if you give the right answer and some rationale for that answer, it is assumed you were **applying thinking**. Students typically explain their thinking only in terms of content, not in terms of thinking; therefore, there is no evidence that **applying thinking** actually occurred.

Now that you have studied Section I, you are beginning to understand what clinical judgment actually is. Clinical judgment is an actual process you learn and use when working through patient situations and other nursing issues on a healthcare unit. Using the Caputi Clinical Judgment Framework prepares you to address new, unfamiliar issues because you have an approach to use to work through the thinking required to address the issue. Using the clinical judgment process is how you address the **apply thinking** part of nursing; however, **applying thinking** doesn't just happen. It must be learned!

Content and clinical judgment (thinking) MUST go together; otherwise, there is no assurance your thinking will lead to the best results. Therefore, explaining your thinking by only addressing content is not actually explaining your thinking. Explaining your thinking is two-dimensional:

1. **CONTENT** ~ Explaining the content that relates to what you are thinking including pathophysiology; patient health information; patient-specific information such as spirituality, culture, and pre-existing conditions; medications and other treatments the patient is receiving; interventions you planned; rationales for your interventions; nursing interventions you performed; how the patient responded; and other information relevant to the patient and the discussion. All this is the **content** you learn in your nursing courses and associate with, or connect to, an individual patient situation.

2. **CLINICAL JUDGMENT** ~ Explaining your thinking. The content is central to what you are doing as a nurse (situation-based thinking); however, the content takes on true meaning only if you can explain how you used that content in terms of the organized **thinking** you used. You must explain **how your thinking guided** your use of the content.

The clinical judgment piece of the NCLEX beginning in Spring, 2023 requires the candidate to apply clinical judgment as needed. The activities in Section II (Chapters 8 and 9) give you practice doing just that. All these **Advanced Level Cognitive Guidance Tools** require you to use the clinical judgment competencies of the Caputi Clinical Judgment Framework that provide the basis for the clinical judgment tested on the Next Generation NCLEX. Recall Table 1 previously presented in Chapter 1.

TABLE 1

How the Caputi Clinical Judgment Framework Supports the Thinking of the NCLEX Clinical Judgment Measurement Model

The Cognitive Processes of the NCLEX NGN Clinical Judgment Measurement Model	Major Steps in the Caputi Clinical Judgment Framework	The Caputi Clinical Judgment Competencies Used with Each of the Six Cognitive Processes of the NGN
1. Recognize Cues	Getting the Information	• Determining important information to collect • Scanning the environment • Identifying signs and symptoms • Assessing systematically and comprehensively • Ensuring accurate information
2. Analyze Cues	Making Meaning of the Information	• Clustering related information • Identifying assumptions • Recognizing inconsistencies • Distinguishing relevant from irrelevant information • Judging how much ambiguity is acceptable • Comparing and contrasting • Predicting potential complications • Collaborating with healthcare team members • Determining patient care needs/ healthcare environment issues
3. Prioritize Hypotheses	Determining Actions to Take	• Setting priorities
4. Generate Solutions	Determining Actions to Take	• Selecting interventions • Managing potential complications
5. Take Actions	Taking Action	• Determining how to implement the planned interventions • Delegating • Communicating • Teaching others
6. Evaluate Outcomes	Evaluating Outcomes and Your Thinking	• Evaluating data • Evaluating and correcting thinking

Practice applying and **explaining** how you use the various clinical judgment competencies prepares you for the Next Generation NCLEX because you have learned how to think using the six cognitive processes of the NCSBN's Clinical Judgment Measurement Model.

Section II (Chapters 8 and 9) provides many activities for you to apply the Caputi Clinical Judgment Framework when caring for patients and when faced with other nursing concerns that are not patient related. In Section I each of the cognitive guidance tools was categorized according to a clinical judgment competency. In Section II, the cognitive guidance tools are more complex and **require the use of a number of clinical judgment competencies**. Therefore, most of the tools are not categorized according to a clinical judgment competency, but require you to determine what thinking from the clinical judgment framework is needed to complete the activity. The few tools that are named using a clinical judgment competency are more complex tools than the ones presented in Chapters 3 through 7. Once you finish the tool you will complete a table listing each of the clinical judgment competencies to explain which of the clinical judgment competencies you used and how you used each one.

These more complex activities move you from focusing on a particular clinical judgment competency to focusing on application of the entire framework of thinking, using whichever clinical judgment competencies are required to complete the task. Completing the "Table to Explain Your Thinking" located at the end of Chapters 8 and 9 is very important because it requires you to **reflect** on your thinking. This reflection is critical to your growth in the use of clinical judgment.

Using the Advanced Level Cognitive Guidance Tools in Chapters 8 and 9 is the bridge that connects learning each of the clinical judgment competencies to becoming a self-directed thinker who automatically applies the Caputi Clinical Judgment Framework in new nursing situations.

Content and clinical judgment (thinking) MUST go together; otherwise, there is no assurance your thinking will lead to the best results.

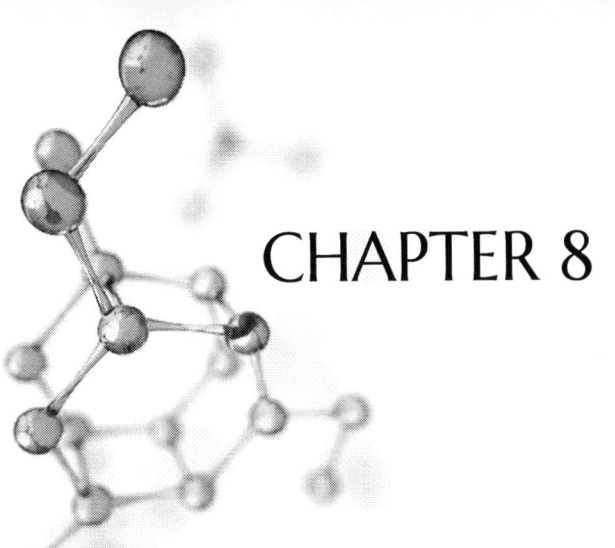

CHAPTER 8

Advanced Level Cognitive Guidance Tools

AS YOU LEARNED IN THE first seven chapters of this book, nurses use clinical judgment continuously throughout the day, although their thinking is not visually evident. As a student you must assume the nurse is thinking, yet you can't "see" the thinking. You learned how nurses think by learning all the clinical judgment competencies then practiced using them with real patients in the clinical setting. The clinical setting is the primary place to sharpen your skills of clinical judgment. The practice part of learning clinical judgment can be difficult, but is one of the most critical elements to learn how to think like a nurse.

This chapter provides Advanced Cognitive Guidance Tools for you to use in the clinical setting after the first term (semester, quarter, or whatever system is used at your school) when you used the cognitive tools in Chapters 3 through 7.

The activities you will engage in when using the tools in Chapters 8 and 9 are different from the ones you used in Chapters 3 through 7 in a few important ways.

1. These activities are not labeled with a specific clinical judgment competency or a step in the Caputi Clinical Judgment Framework.

2. These activities require an in-depth look at a situation with application of several (or many) clinical judgment competencies.

3. After you complete the activity, you will explain which clinical judgment competencies you used to complete the

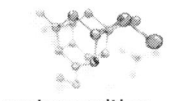

metacognition ~

the ability to analyze and explain your own thinking

activity. You will then explain how you used each clinical judgment competency to complete the activity. This analysis of your own thinking is called metacognition. Metacognition refers to your ability to explain your thinking. Engaging in metacognition means you understand, analyze, and control your own cognitive processes. The Caputi Clinical Judgment Competencies provide the language you can use to explain your thinking. Practice explaining your thinking is a necessary activity for you to complete as you continue on your path to becoming a self-directed thinker. As discussed in Chapter 1, this is one of the overall reasons for learning clinical judgment—to become a self-directed thinker.

Consult with your faculty to determine when you'll use these tools in your clinical experience. If you don't use some of the tools in your clinical experience, you may reflect on patients for whom you have cared and think about how you would have worked through that thinking activity based on that patient's situation.

As your abilities in nursing practice develop with the use of the Caputi Clinical Judgment Framework, so will your ability to use the clinical judgment competencies to explain your thinking. The nurse who is able to engage in, be aware of, and explain use of these higher levels of thinking is better prepared to provide safe, quality patient care and improve patient outcomes.

CHAPTER 8 ■ Advanced Level Cognitive Guidance Tools 217

ADVANCED COGNITIVE GUIDANCE TOOL

WHAT WOULD YOU DO DIFFERENTLY?

As a nurse, you collect lots of patient information. "Getting the Information" is the first step of the Caputi Clinical Judgment Framework. Some of the information is used to "Evaluate Outcomes" when the nurse engages in the clinical judgment competencies of Step 2: "Making Meaning of the Information" and the clinical judgment competency of *Evaluating Data*. This thinking directly relates to the NCSBN's Clinical Judgment cognitive processes of "Analyzing Cues" and "Evaluating Outcomes."

To complete Table 8.1, assess your patient and review the assessment data collected over the last 24 hours. Use that information to complete Table 8.1.

TABLE 8.1

What Would You Do Differently?

Time When the Data Were Collected	Assessment Data Over the Last 24 Hours (Including Your Own Assessment at this Time)	Nursing Interventions/ Actions Related to Assessment Data	Why the Nursing Actions were Taken (Include Patient Data to Substantiate Your Rationale)	What You Would Do Differently and Why

Add more rows as needed

Explaining Your Use of the Clinical Judgment Competencies

What clinical judgment competencies did you use? Complete Table 8.17 at the end of this chapter explaining which clinical judgment competencies you used and how you used each one to complete the activity.

ADVANCED COGNITIVE GUIDANCE TOOL

WORSE, BETTER, OR NOT RELATED?

This Advanced Level Cognitive Guidance Tool is similar to the previous one, but a little different. This tool requires you to make a determination about the care provided based on the data you collect.

Assess your patient and review the assessment data collected over the last 12 to 24 hours. Use that information to complete Table 8.2.

TABLE 8.2

Worse, Better, or Not Related?

Patient Assessment Data at Current Time	Same Assessment 12 Hours Earlier	Same Assessment 24 Hours Earlier	Does the Current Assessment Data Indicate the Patient is Better/Worse Or... The Data are Not Related to the Medical Diagnosis *Explain*

Add more rows as needed

Explaining Your Use of the Clinical Judgment Competencies

What clinical judgment competencies did you use? Complete Table 8.17 at the end of this chapter explaining which clinical judgment competencies you used and how you used each one to complete the activity.

CHAPTER 8 ■ Advanced Level Cognitive Guidance Tools

ADVANCED COGNITIVE GUIDANCE TOOL

WHAT TO DO WHEN?

This Advanced Level Cognitive Guidance Tool continues to focus on patient assessment data. This tool requires you to determine what information needs immediate attention and actions you will take.

Assess your patient and review the assessment data collected over the last 12 hours. Use that information to complete Table 8.3.

TABLE 8.3

What To Do When?

Patient Assessment Data at Current Time	Same Assessment 12 Hours Earlier	Determine Which Assessment Data to Address (Needs Immediate Attention) Explain	What Actions Will You Take to Address the Immediate Needs?

Add more rows as needed

Explaining Your Use of the Clinical Judgment Competencies

What clinical judgment competencies did you use? Complete Table 8.17 at the end of this chapter explaining which clinical judgment competencies you used and how you used each one to complete the activity.

ADVANCED COGNITIVE GUIDANCE TOOL

EFFECTIVE, INEFFECTIVE, OR UNRELATED?

This Advanced Level Cognitive Guidance Tool continues to focus on patient assessment data. This tool requires you to determine the effectiveness of nursing interventions.

Assess your patient and review the assessment data collected over the last 12 to 24 hours. Relate the assessment data to the nursing interventions implemented. Use that information to complete Table 8.4.

TABLE 8.4

Effective, Ineffective, or Unrelated?

Patient Assessment Data at Current Time and Entries on Previous Nurse's Documentation About Those Same Assessments	Nursing Interventions Implemented	Based on the Assessment Data and Nurses' Notes, Was the Intervention Effective, Ineffective, or Unrelated?	What Actions Will You Take for the Interventions You Determine are Ineffective?

Add more rows as needed

Explaining Your Use of the Clinical Judgment Competencies

What clinical judgment competencies did you use? Complete Table 8.17 at the end of this chapter explaining which clinical judgment competencies you used and how you used each one to complete the activity.

ADVANCED COGNITIVE GUIDANCE TOOL

DETERMINING NURSING INTERVENTIONS BASED ON SIGNS AND SYMPTOMS

In addition to all the patient-specific information the nurse uses when planning patient care, the pathophysiology of any disease the patient is experiencing is also important when planning nursing interventions. Various clinical judgment competencies are applied to determine what nursing actions to implement for the individual patient related to the patient's unique, individual experience with the disease(s).

Study your patient's various medical diagnoses. Assess your patient for data related to those medical diagnoses, including any diagnostic results or other information in the patient's medical record. Relate the data to nursing interventions to implement.
Use that information to complete Table 8.5.

TABLE 8.5
Determining Nursing Interventions

Medical Diagnoses Including Pre-existing Diseases	Signs & Symptoms of the Diagnoses Based on the Pathophysiology	Signs and Symptoms this Patient is Manifesting	Nursing Actions to Take Related to the Individual Patient's Manifestations

Add more rows as needed

Explaining Your Use of the Clinical Judgment Competencies

What clinical judgment competencies did you use? Complete Table 8.17 at the end of this chapter explaining which clinical judgment competencies you used and how you used each one to complete the activity.

ADVANCED COGNITIVE GUIDANCE TOOL

PLANNING SAFE CARE

Nurses plan safe care by "Determining Actions to Take" based on the patient information collected and analyzed. In addition to planning nursing interventions, the nurse anticipates what other providers may order. The nurse also ensures that other nursing personnel taking care of the patient only provide care that will benefit, not harm, the patient. For that reason, the nurse anticipates what other healthcare providers may order but also considers what actions NOT to take to ensure no harm comes to the patient.

After you assess your patient, complete Table 8.6.

TABLE 8.6
Determining Care to Provide

Patient Assessment Data at Current Time	What physician or primary healthcare provider orders do you anticipate receiving?	What nursing interventions will you implement?	What nursing interventions would be CONTRAINDICATED or HARMFUL for this patient?

Add more rows as needed

Explaining Your Use of the Clinical Judgment Competencies

What clinical judgment competencies did you use? Complete Table 8.17 at the end of this chapter explaining which clinical judgment competencies you used and how you used each one to complete the activity.

ADVANCED COGNITIVE GUIDANCE TOOL

PAIN ASSESSMENT

A cognitive guidance tool focused on pain assessment was provided in Chapter 3, Table 3.5 in this book when studying the clinical judgment competency of *Assessing Systematically and Comprehensively*. This tool is again presented in Table 8.7. In this Advanced Level Cognitive Guidance Tool, you will collect data from three different patients. You examine the results of your assessment of three patients and identify differences or nuances. Although some differences or nuances may be subtle, they may influence the actions the nurse takes when planning individualized, patient-centered care. It is important to identify these differences to ensure individualized, situation-based care.

TABLE 8.7

Pain Assessment Tool

Pain Assessment Component	Data Collection
O ~ Onset	When did the pain start?
P ~ Palliation/Provocation	What makes the pain better? Worse?
Q ~ Quality	What does the pain feel like (sharp, dull, stabbing, burning)?
R ~ Region/Radiation	Where is your pain? Does it radiate/move anywhere else?
S ~ Severity	Rate your pain on a numeric rating scale (NRS) 0 to 10, with 0 being no pain and 10 being the worst pain possible (rate at rest and with activity)
T ~ Timing	Is the pain constant or intermittent? How long does it last?
U ~ Understanding	What do you believe is causing the pain? How is the pain impacting you? Your family? The patient's perception of pain and what the pain means to the patient.
V ~ Value	What is an acceptable level for this pain (NRS 0-10)? Any other symptoms related to the pain? Anything else you would like to say about your pain?
Other factors	Explore other factors which may influence the pain response (culture, past pain experiences, medical history related to pain)

TABLE 8.7 *(continued)*

Pain Assessment Tool

Pain Assessment Component	Data Collection
Pain Behaviors (verbal and non-verbal pain indicators)	Verbal expressions of pain. Non-verbal indicators of pain (facial features, body, muscle tension, moaning, crying, others)
Affective Responses	Signs of anxiety, depression, patterns of interacting with others, effect of pain on ability to perform daily activities, adaptive mechanism to cope with the pain
Medications	Medication and dose the patient is taking for pain
	Frequency taking the medication
	Patient's pain score prior to receiving the medication and pain score 30 minutes after receiving the medication
	The patient's evaluation/perception of the effectiveness of the medication
	Any side effects or untoward effects the patient is experiencing
Non-Medication Relief Measures	What non-medication relief measures are provided to the patient (heat/cold application, positioning, relaxation, distraction, acupuncture, other)?
	Patient's evaluation of the effectiveness of the relief measures
Other Data	Note additional important information about the patient and the patient's pain not included in the above
	Note physiologic responses such as vital signs, perspiration, pupil size, nausea, muscle tension, anxiety

Analyze the data for each of the three patients, then answer the following questions:

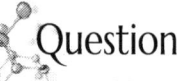

Question

How is each patient responding to the treatment for pain?

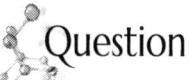

Question

What factors are most influential for each of the patient's control of pain?

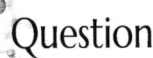
Question

Compare the medications for each patient. How are they the same? How are they different?

Question

Why do different patients receive different pain medications?

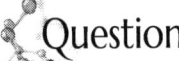
Question

What are some conclusions you can make about the differences among these three patients and how those differences influence the care the nurse will provide?

Explaining Your Use of the Clinical Judgment Competencies

What clinical judgment competencies did you use? Complete Table 8.17 at the end of this chapter explaining which clinical judgment competencies you used and how you used each one to complete the activity.

ADVANCED COGNITIVE GUIDANCE TOOL

PREDICTING AND MANAGING POTENTIAL COMPLICATIONS

These two clinical judgment competencies are combined in this Advanced Level Cognitive Guidance Tool. The purpose is to demonstrate the critical connection between the two. Other clinical judgment competencies are used when working through the thinking for *Predicting and Managing Potential Complications*.

Complete this tool for the patient you are assigned or use it to assess three patients. If using with three patients, you may work with another student if approved by your faculty.

Answer the following questions for each patient:

Question

What are you on alert for today with this patient?

Explain why this is important.

Question

What are the important assessments to make?

Explain why these assessments are important.

Question

For each of the important assessments to make, what parameters will you apply for each?

Explain how you determined the upper and lower limits of the parameters.

Question

What complications may occur? What could go wrong?

Relate the assessment data to the potential complications that may occur.

Question
How will you know if a complication is actually occurring?

Question
What interventions will prevent each complication from occurring?

Discuss how the interventions prevent complications.

Question
What will you do if the complication does occur?

Explain how your planned interventions immediately treat, stop, or reverse the complication.

Discuss
What puts each patient at risk for the complication identified?

Discuss
If completing the tool for three patients, why are there differences among the three patients?

Explaining Your Use of the Clinical Judgment Competencies

What clinical judgment competencies did you use? Complete Table 8.17 at the end of this chapter explaining which clinical judgment competencies you used and how you used each one to complete the activity.

ADVANCED COGNITIVE GUIDANCE TOOL

NATIONAL PATIENT SAFETY GOALS

The National Patient Safety Goals (NPSGs) are a standard for ensuring basic safety for patients in a variety of healthcare environments. Access the NPSGs for the healthcare environment in which you are working. These are available at: www.jointcommission.org/standards_information/npsgs.aspx

Using the NPSGs as a guide, answer the following questions for each patient:

Question
What precautions should you take relative to each safety goal for your patient?

Question
For your patient, is there a safety goal that is most relevant? Explain how and why you determined which was most important.

Question
What factors about the environment indicate the safety goals are being met?

Question
What factors about the environment indicate a need for change so the safety goals can be met?

Question
How will you incorporate knowledge of the NPSGs into your practice as a nurse?

Explaining Your Use of the Clinical Judgment Competencies

What clinical judgment competencies did you use? Complete Table 8.17 at the end of this chapter explaining which clinical judgment competencies you used and how you used each one to complete the activity.

ADVANCED COGNITIVE GUIDANCE TOOL

APPLYING CLINICAL JUDGMENT TO PERFORMING NURSING SKILLS

A list of steps, called a checklist, is typically used when teaching/learning a specific nursing psychomotor skill. Novice nurses use that checklist to ensure all steps of the procedure are performed. As the nurse's ability to consider each patient as an individual develops, it becomes apparent the specific order and approach to each step for performing a nursing skill may need to be modified for a particular patient. This Advanced Level Cognitive Guidance Tool requires you to consider information about a patient situation that is used to determine how a particular nursing skill is performed.

This activity requires you to reference a nursing skills checklist for a skill of your choice. This checklist can be for a nursing skill that in some way relates to your patient. It does not need to be for a nursing skill you will actually perform. For example, your patient does not have a healthcare provider's order for insertion of a retention urinary catheter, but you may still use a checklist for this procedure and work through the activity as though an order is in place.

Review the skills checklist you selected. Visit your patient and perform a head-to-assessment.

Answer the following questions:

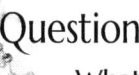
Question
What information did you gather during the assessment that is important to consider when preparing to perform the skill? Explain.

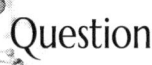
Question
Which data are relevant to the performance of the skill; that is, which data require you to modify **the order of the steps** of the skill as they are written? Explain.

Question

Which data require you **to modify the manner** in which any of the steps of the skill are performed?

Explain.

Question

What precautions will you take to ensure the skill is performed with the modified approach without compromising patient safety?

Explain.

Explaining Your Use of the Clinical Judgment Competencies

What clinical judgment competencies did you use? Complete Table 8.17 at the end of this chapter explaining which clinical judgment competencies you used and how you used each one to complete the activity.

ADVANCED COGNITIVE GUIDANCE TOOL

RELEVANT DATA ON WHICH TO ACT

In every patient situation, there are numerous pieces of information to sort through. Sorting through the information can be a bit of a challenge when working through case studies in class or through a simulation experience. However, in the real-world of nursing you encounter in the clinical setting, the information may seem endless. The nurse must sort through the seemingly endless amount of patient information and focus on that which is most important for that patient and relevant to the identified issues or concerns.

Review your patient's history and perform a patient assessment. Select the activity below which aligns with your patient.

Patient Treated Surgically (either scheduled for surgery or is postoperative)
Read the patient's history and physical, including previous surgeries, medical history, and medications taken prior to admission. Discuss which information from the review of the patient's medical record and your assessment will have an impact on the patient's recovery from surgery. Be sure to identify (1) what might interfere with the patient's recovery from surgery, and (2) what will benefit the patient's recovery and why. For each piece of information determine which data will most influence the care you will provide this day.

Patient Being Treated Medically
For your patient being treated medically for an illness, discuss which information from the review of the patient's medical record and your assessment will have an impact on the patient's recovery from the current illness. Be sure to identify (1) what might interfere with the patient's recovery from the illness, and (2) what will benefit the patient's recovery and why. For each piece of information determine which data are relevant to the care you will provide this day.

Explaining Your Use of the Clinical Judgment Competencies
What clinical judgment competencies did you use? Complete Table 8.17 at the end of this chapter explaining which clinical judgment competencies you used and how you used each one to complete the activity.

ADVANCED COGNITIVE GUIDANCE TOOL

WHAT TO DO WITH DATA

This Advanced Level Cognitive Guidance Tool provides practice with processing patient data. Nurses collect a lot of patient data; safe patient care requires knowing what to do with all that data. Nurses must determine what data to act on and what data do not require action.

Perform a patient assessment.
After your assessment, answer the following questions.

Question
What patient data did you collect?

Question
What data are out of range?

Question
What further data did/should you collect?

Question
What will you do with that data?

Question
How will you use the additional data you decided to collect in order to make a decision about the original assessment data?

Question
What parameters (high and low readings) will you apply about the data under consideration that will call you to action? That is, what readings related to the data require a nursing action?

CHAPTER 8 ■ Advanced Level Cognitive Guidance Tools   233

*After completing the above questions,
answer the following questions.*

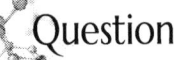
Question
What decisions did you make and why?

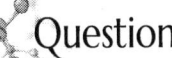
Question
What is the basis for your decisions?

Question
What will you do next and why?

Explaining Your Use of the Clinical Judgment Competencies

What clinical judgment competencies did you use? Complete Table 8.17 at the end of this chapter explaining which clinical judgment competencies you used and how you used each one to complete the activity.

ADVANCED COGNITIVE GUIDANCE TOOL

PLANNING PATIENT CARE

Read about your patient's condition in a nursing textbook or other reference. List the nursing interventions as recommended in the nursing textbook or other reference.

Complete Table 8.8.

TABLE 8.8

Planning Patient Care

Interventions Based on the Textbook	Indicated for this Patient? Why or why not?	Modifications You Will Make to the Textbook Plan of Care

Add additional rows as needed

Explaining Your Use of the Clinical Judgment Competencies

What clinical judgment competencies did you use? Complete Table 8.17 at the end of this chapter explaining which clinical judgment competencies you used and how you used each one to complete the activity.

ADVANCED COGNITIVE GUIDANCE TOOL

COMPARING AND CONTRASTING THREE PATIENTS WITH THE SAME MEDICAL DIAGNOSIS

Select three patients with the same medical diagnosis (for example, same surgical procedure, same medical condition, same healthcare issue such as dementia). Using the electronic medical record, collect the following information on all three patients. If approved by your faculty, you may work with another student on this activity.

- History

- Current medical diagnosis

- Other pre-existing conditions

- Diet

- Medications

- Treatments

- Limitations in function

- Medical procedure(s) performed

- Other relevant information

Complete Table 8.9 for each patient.
Be sure to discuss variations noted and reasons why diet, meds, treatments, etc.,
are different among the three patients.

TABLE 8.9

Comparing and Contrasting Three Patients ~ PATIENT #1

PATIENT #1: Data Collected	How the data are the same/different from the other patients
History:	
Current medical diagnosis:	
Other pre-existing conditions:	
Diet:	
Medications:	
Treatment:	
Limitations in function:	
Procedures performed:	
Other relevant information:	

TABLE 8.9 *(continued)*

Comparing and Contrasting Three Patients ~ PATIENT #2

PATIENT #2: Data Collected	How the data are the same/different from the other patients
History:	
Current medical diagnosis:	
Other pre-existing conditions:	
Diet:	
Medications:	
Treatment:	
Limitations in function:	
Procedures performed:	
Other relevant information:	

TABLE 8.9 *(continued)*

Comparing and Contrasting Three Patients ~ PATIENT #3

PATIENT #3: Data Collected	How the data are the same/different from the other patients
History:	
Current medical diagnosis:	
Other pre-existing conditions:	
Diet:	
Medications:	
Treatment:	
Limitations in function:	
Procedures performed:	
Other relevant information:	

Complete Table 8.10.
Review all the data for each patient and note which findings are out of range
and what actions are needed. Note potential complications for each patient
and nursing interventions to prevent those complications.

TABLE 8.10

Identifying Possible Complications

Patient	Specific findings that are out of range	Actions to take	Potential complications	Interventions to prevent those complications
#1				
#2				
#3				

Explaining Your Use of the Clinical Judgment Competencies

What clinical judgment competencies did you use? Complete Table 8.17 at the end of this chapter explaining which clinical judgment competencies you used and how you used each one to complete the activity.

ADVANCED COGNITIVE GUIDANCE TOOL

SETTING PRIORITIES

This Advanced Level Cognitive Guidance Tool offers a different approach for the clinical judgment competency of *Setting Priorities* than was presented in Chapter 5. It is important to realize there are a number of ways to prioritize care; the nurse determines the best approach based on the individual patient's needs.

After assessing your patient, list the needs the patient has at this time and categorize the identified patient needs using the following criteria in the space below. Explain your rationale.

1. First order priority need—immediate threat to health, safety, or survival

2. Second order priority need—actual problem for which immediate help has been requested by the patient or family

3. Third order priority need—actual or potential issue about which the patient or family is not aware

4. Fourth order priority need—actual or potential issue that is anticipated in the future and for which help will be needed

First Order Priority Needs with Rationale—

Second Order Priority Needs with Rationale—

Third Order Priority Needs with Rationale—

Fourth Order Priority Needs with Rationale—

Explaining Your Use of the Clinical Judgment Competencies

What clinical judgment competencies did you use? Complete Table 8.17 at the end of this chapter explaining which clinical judgment competencies you used and how you used each one to complete the activity.

ADVANCED COGNITIVE GUIDANCE TOOL

TEACHING OTHERS

This Advanced Level Cognitive Guidance Tool focuses on discharge teaching. Consider all the information you collected about your patient.

Complete Table 8.11.

TABLE 8.11

Teaching Others

Important information to include in discharge teaching	Why this information is important	How you obtained the information	What you will teach about this information	Method(s) used to teach the information

Add additional rows as needed

Once your teaching is complete, evaluate your teaching.

Answer the following questions.

Question

Did the patient/family/significant other understand what you were teaching? Explain how you know; what is the evidence?

Question

Was the patient/family/significant other able to demonstrate that learning occurred? How do you know?

Question

Is there a need to work at a later time with the patient/family/significant other to reinforce what was taught? Explain.

Explaining Your Use of the Clinical Judgment Competencies

What clinical judgment competencies did you use? Complete Table 8.17 at the end of this chapter explaining which clinical judgment competencies you used and how you used each one to complete the activity.

ADVANCED COGNITIVE GUIDANCE TOOL

USING CLINICAL JUDGMENT COMPETENCIES TO COMPLETE THE SBAR FORM

Some version of SBAR is used in most healthcare institutions. Completing the SBAR is not a task of "filling in the blanks." The information the nurse includes in each section of the report is determined only after applying clinical judgment competencies.

This activity requires you to analyze the thinking you use to determine the data to include in your SBAR report. Table 8.12 uses the SBAR version minus the "I" as in the version presented in Chapters 4 and 6. The "I" would not be used if you are using this tool to directly communicate with someone face-to-face. Using Table 8.12 explain how you used each clinical judgment competency (CJC) and the information that resulted from application of the clinical judgment competencies.

TABLE 8.12

Applying Clinical Judgment to SBAR

S ~ SITUATION:	
Include basic demographics about your patient: name, ethnicity, age, gender, and **relevant information about the patient's condition/situation.** Include patient preferences when appropriate.	1. How did you use each of the following clinical judgment competencies (CJCs) to determine what information to include as "relevant information?" • *Determining important information to collect* • *Identifying signs and symptoms* • *Assessing systematically and comprehensively* • *Distinguishing relevant from irrelevant information* • *Judging how much ambiguity is acceptable* 2. From application of the above CJCs, list the "relevant information about the patient's condition/situation" to include in this section of the SBAR form.

TABLE 8.12 *(continued)*

Applying Clinical Judgment to SBAR

B ~ BACKGROUND: Patient's admitting diagnosis, hospital day, medical history that **might complicate the current admission, any data about what has led up to any issues the patient is currently experiencing.**	1. How did you use each of the following clinical judgment competencies to determine what information to include as "...might complicate the current admission, any data about what has led up to any issues the patient is currently experiencing?" • *Distinguishing relevant from irrelevant information* • *Judging how much ambiguity is acceptable* • *Predicting potential complications* 2. From application of the above CJCs, list information that "...might complicate the current admission, any data about what has led up to any issues the patient is currently experiencing" to include in this section of the SBAR form.
A ~ ASSESSMENT: **Signs and symptoms** related to the issue, including vital signs, O₂ Sats, and **any other relevant assessment data.**	1. How did you use each of the following clinical judgment competencies (CJCs) to determine what information to include as "signs and symptoms" and "other relevant assessment data?" • *Identifying signs and symptoms* • *Assessing systematically and comprehensively* • *Ensuring the information is accurate* • *Recognizing inconsistencies* • *Distinguishing relevant from irrelevant information* 2. From application of the above CJCs, list the "signs and symptoms" and "other relevant assessment data" to include in this section of the SBAR form.
R ~ RECOMMENDATIONS: Include what you have done, the patient's response, suggest what might be needed, request further direction.	1. How did you use each of the following clinical judgment competencies (CJCs) to determine what information to include as "what you have done and the patient's response?" • *Selecting interventions* • *Managing potential complications* • *Setting priorities* • *Evaluating data* 2. From application of the above CJCs, list the "what you have done and the patient's response" to include in this section of the SBAR form.

Explaining Your Use of the Clinical Judgment Competencies

What clinical judgment competencies did you use? Complete Table 8.17 at the end of this chapter explaining which clinical judgment competencies you used and how you used each one to complete the activity.

> **Note**
>
> There is no universal SBAR format used in practice. Each healthcare organization chooses which format to adopt. In addition to the two versions presented in this book (**ISBAR** and **SBAR**), you may encounter others, such as **ISBAR-RQ** which stands for Identify, Situation, Background, Assessment, Recommendation, Read back, and Questions.

ADVANCED COGNITIVE GUIDANCE TOOL

EVALUATING DATA

For this activity answer the following questions.

- What evaluation data will you (did you) collect for each intervention in the patient's plan of care?

- What changes to patient care will you (did you) make based on the evaluation data?

- What findings will trigger you to take immediate action? Explain why and what actions you will take.

Using the answers to the above questions, complete Table 8.13 while caring for your patient throughout the day.

TABLE 8.13

Analyzing Evaluation Data

Which evaluation data indicate the patient's condition is improving? *Explain.*	Which evaluation data indicate the patient's condition is staying the same? *Explain.*	Which evaluation data indicate the patient's condition is declining? *Explain.*

Add additional rows as needed

Explaining Your Use of the Clinical Judgment Competencies

What clinical judgment competencies did you use? Complete Table 8.17 at the end of this chapter explaining which clinical judgment competencies you used and how you used each one to complete the activity.

CHAPTER 8 ■ Advanced Level Cognitive Guidance Tools 247

ADVANCED COGNITIVE GUIDANCE TOOL

EVALUATING AND CORRECTING THINKING

Consider the care you provided today.
Complete the below tool with the requested information or answers to the questions.

Question
Describe one patient issue you identified.

Question
Explain what you did about that issue.

Question
What was the outcome related to the action you took and was that outcome what you expected? Explain.

Question
If the expected outcome was not achieved, what will you do differently?

Question
How did your thinking impact others? Explain.

Question
Was the impact of your thinking positive or negative? Explain.

Explaining Your Use of the Clinical Judgment Competencies

What clinical judgment competencies did you use? Complete Table 8.17 at the end of this chapter explaining which clinical judgment competencies you used and how you used each one to complete the activity.

ADVANCED COGNITIVE GUIDANCE TOOL

SAFETY AND MEDICATION ADMINISTRATION

Safe administration of medications involves much more than the act of administering the medication to the patient. There is much information a nurse uses prior to, during, and after administering medications to the patient. This Advanced Level Cognitive Guidance Tool explores the information used by the nurse to safely administer medications.

Gather the following information

- Patient's medical diagnosis
- Allergies
- Surgical or other procedure
- Chronic conditions

Consider information about the medication and how it relates to the patient

- Medication to be administered
- Classification of the medication
- Reason why the medication is prescribed for this patient
- How this medication relates to the patient's history and physical
- Other prescribed medications that affect the administration of this medication
- Expected therapeutic effect(s)
- Side effects to consider
- The effects of the medication the last time it was given

Determine how to safely administer the medication

- Patient identification
- Relevant assessments to make
- Parameters to consider
- Contraindications to administering this medication
- Reasons to hold (not administer) this medication
- Dosage that will be administered
- Route that will be used
- IV medications:
  - ~ Compatible with IV solution?
  - ~ Medication compatible with other meds in the line
  - ~ Flush needed?
  - ~ Explain compatibility between this medication and others being administered.

- Oral medication:
  - ~ Can it be crushed?
  - ~ Given with food?
  - ~ Can it be given with other medications? Explain.

- Injectable medications:
  - ~ Factors to consider when choosing the right site?
  - ~ Special considerations for the ordered medication?
  - ~ How to ensure injection safety for self? Patient?

Explaining Your Use of the Clinical Judgment Competencies

What clinical judgment competencies did you use? Complete Table 8.17 at the end of this chapter explaining which clinical judgment competencies you used and how you used each one to complete the activity.

ADVANCED COGNITIVE GUIDANCE TOOL

DELEGATING AND SETTING PRIORITIES

This Advanced Level Cognitive Guidance Tool combines the two clinical judgment competencies of *Delegating* and *Setting Priorities*.

Today you have the following team members working with you; an LPN/VN and a nursing assistant. Collect the following information about your patient as well as two other patients. If approved by your faculty, you may work with another student on this activity.

- **Medical Diagnosis**
- **Nursing care for today**
    - ~ Activity level and assistance needed with activity
    - ~ Diet and assistance needed to eat or special needs related to nutrition
    - ~ Nursing procedures: dressing changes, suctioning, others
    - ~ Intravenous therapy (fluid, rate)
    - ~ State of fluid balance (include assessments you made to determine fluid balance)
    - ~ Patient teaching
    - ~ Other nursing care and treatments the nurse will perform
- **Pain**
    - ~ Pain rating
    - ~ Medications ordered for pain
    - ~ Side effects of analgesics to consider
- **Safety issues for this patient**
- **Labs scheduled for today and how the labs relate to nursing care**
- **Other diagnostic studies scheduled for today and how the studies relate to nursing care**
- **Medications**
    - ~ Classification of the medication
    - ~ Reasons why the medication is ordered for this patient
    - ~ Schedule for administering the medication
    - ~ Patient teaching relative to the medication
    - ~ Any special instructions regarding administration of this medication
    - ~ Which medication for each patient is most important to administer on time and why?
    - ~ What might happen if the medication is not administered on time?

CHAPTER 8 ■ Advanced Level Cognitive Guidance Tools 251

Visit each patient and perform a two-minute assessment of both the patient and the patient's environment.

Answer the following questions based on the information you collected.

Question
Prioritize which patient you should care for first, second, and third. Explain.

Question
What are the primary assessments to complete first for each patient? Explain.

Question
What nursing interventions need to be carried out for each patient?

Question
What interventions will you do first? Explain.

Question
Which of the above interventions can be delegated and to whom? Explain.

Question
What information will be given to the person to whom the task is delegated and what information will be collected after the task is complete?

Explaining Your Use of the Clinical Judgment Competencies

What clinical judgment competencies did you use? Complete Table 8.17 at the end of this chapter explaining which clinical judgment competencies you used and how you used each one to complete the activity.

ADVANCED COGNITIVE GUIDANCE TOOL

CALLING THE PHYSICIAN OR OTHER PRIMARY HEALTHCARE PROVIDER (PHCP)

When using the clinical judgment competencies of *Communicating* and *Collaborating with Healthcare Team Members*, the SBAR format is often used. However, completion of the SBAR form first requires the nurse to apply clinical judgment competencies to determine what to include on the SBAR form.

The Advanced Level Cognitive Guidance Tool in Table 8.14 helps you determine how to implement the Caputi Clinical Judgment Framework for better communication and collaboration.

Answer the following questions.

Question
What led you to believe you need to call the physician or other PHCP? Explain.

Question
Have you formulated a clear picture of the problem? What is it?

Question
Have you read the most recent MD/PHCP progress notes and notes from the nurse on the previous shift? What information is relevant to this situation? Explain.

Question
Should you discuss the issue with the charge nurse before calling? Why or why not?

Question
What do you expect to happen as a result of this call? Explain.

Question

What information do you need to collect before you call the physician/PHCP?

Question

When calling, remember that part of communicating is to provide identifying information:

a. Identify yourself, unit, patient, room #

b. Include the admitting diagnosis and date of admission

c. Use the completed SBAR form to ensure complete, accurate communication

TABLE 8.14

Communicating with the Primary Healthcare Provider

S ~ SITUATION: Include basic demographics about your patient: name, ethnicity, age, gender, and **relevant information about the patient's condition/situation.** Include patient preferences when appropriate.	
B ~ BACKGROUND: Patient's admitting diagnosis, hospital day, medical history that **might complicate the current admission, any data about what has led up to any issues the patient is currently experiencing.**	

TABLE 8.14 (continued)

Communicating with the Primary Healthcare Provider

A ~ ASSESSMENT: Signs and symptoms related to the issue, including vital signs, O₂ Sats, and any other relevant assessment data.	
R ~ RECOMMENDATIONS: Include what you have done, the patient's response, suggest what might be needed, request further direction..	

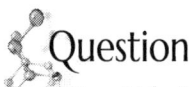

Question

What will you need to document after the call?

Explaining Your Use of the Clinical Judgment Competencies

What clinical judgment competencies did you use? Complete Table 8.17 at the end of this chapter explaining which clinical judgment competencies you used and how you used each one to complete the activity.

ADVANCED COGNITIVE GUIDANCE TOOL

CARING FOR A PATIENT POST-PROCEDURE

Nurses care for patients who have undergone a procedure. Procedures include surgery, an invasive procedure to perform a diagnostic test, and other non-surgical invasive procedures such as a colonoscopy to remove a polyp. Each of these procedures present possible complications. Nurses are alert for possible complications to prevent them, but also to manage them should they occur. If you are caring for a patient undergoing a procedure, you must use clinical forethought to anticipate the needs of the patient. Complete Table 8.15 when caring for a patient undergoing a procedure.

TABLE 8.15

Safe Care of a Patient Undergoing a Procedure

Type of Procedure	Post-Procedure Nursing Care	Possible Potential Post-Procedure Complications	What to Monitor Related to Possible Complications	Nursing Care to Manage Complications Should They Occur

Add more rows as needed

Explaining Your Use of the Clinical Judgment Competencies

What clinical judgment competencies did you use? Complete Table 8.17 at the end of this chapter explaining which clinical judgment competencies you used and how you used each one to complete the activity.

ADVANCED COGNITIVE GUIDANCE TOOL

A QUICK LOOK AT PLANNING PATIENT CARE

Conduct a patient assessment.
Start your planning of patient care by completing Table 8.16.

TABLE 8.16

Planning Patient Care

Questions to Ask	Your Answers
MAKING MEANING OF THE INFORMATION What information is relevant? What information is most important? What information is of immediate concern? Based on the information, what conditions (issues, concerns, possible unidentified medical diagnoses) might the patient be experiencing? What information supports the particular condition you identified? Why are particular pieces of information cause for concern? What additional information would further support the conditions you identified?	
DETERMINING ACTIONS TO TAKE Rank the identified conditions according to urgency or those at highest risk for causing further concern. Which conditions are most likely to worsen if left untreated? What are the desirable outcomes or goals for the identified concerns?	

TABLE 8.16 *(continued)*

Planning Patient Care

Questions to Ask	Your Answers
TAKING ACTION What actions will you take? What actions should be **avoided**? What information is of immediate concern? Based on what you know about the individual patient, what actions will you take and how will you implement them specifically for this patient?	
EVALUATING DATA What is the appropriate time frame to re-assess your patient to determine if the actions were effective? What signs point to the patient improving, declining, or experiencing an unchanged status?	

Explaining Your Use of the Clinical Judgment Competencies

What clinical judgment competencies did you use? Complete Table 8.17 at the end of this chapter explaining which clinical judgment competencies you used and how you used each one to complete the activity.

ADVANCED COGNITIVE GUIDANCE TOOL

TABLE TO EXPLAIN YOUR THINKING

TABLE 8.17

Explaining Your Thinking Using the Caputi Clinical Judgment Framework

Name of Activity: _____

Clinical Judgment Competencies	Which Clinical Judgment Competency Was Used and How it Was Used
Getting the Information 1. Determining important information to collect 2. Scanning the environment 3. Identifying signs and symptoms 4. Assessing systematically and comprehensively 5. Ensuring accurate information	
Making Meaning of the Information 1. Clustering related information 2. Identifying assumptions 3. Recognizing inconsistencies 4. Distinguishing relevant from irrelevant information 5. Judging how much ambiguity is acceptable 6. Comparing and contrasting 7. Predicting potential complications 8. Collaborating with healthcare team members 9. Determining patient care needs/healthcare environment issues	

TABLE 8.17 *(continued)*

Explaining Your Thinking Using the Caputi Clinical Judgment Framework

Clinical Judgment Competencies	Which Clinical Judgment Competency Was Used and How it Was Used
Determining Actions to Take 1. Selecting interventions 2. Managing potential complications 3. Setting priorities	
Taking Action 1. Determining how to implement the planned interventions 2. Delegating (Assigning for some PN/VNs) 3. Communicating 4. Teaching others	
Evaluating Outcomes and Your Thinking 1. Evaluating data 2. Evaluating and correcting thinking	

Chapter 8 Summary

Chapter 8's Advanced Level Cognitive Guidance Tools expand your thinking by requiring you to use many clinical judgment competencies within one activity. These activities require you to use the "Table to Explain Your Thinking" to identify the clinical judgment competencies you used then explain how you used them. This practice, with reflection on your thinking, helps you develop an awareness and understanding of your own thought processes. This is a basic requirement for growing in your ability to engage in clinical judgment. Remember, we don't learn just by having experiences, we learn by reflecting on our experiences. Guided reflection such as that used with the "Table to Explain Your Thinking" helps you process your thinking and learn from your thinking experiences so your thinking will become automatic. This moves you along the path towards becoming a self-directed thinker.

Using the tools in Chapter 8, you explained your thinking in both terms of **content** and **clinical judgment competencies**. The goal of this practice is for you to understand that only using content to explain your thinking does not actually explain your thinking. You must explain your thinking in terms of the clinical judgment competencies you used and how you used them. Being aware of the actual thinking processes you use is what prepares you to deal with new and different situations—ones you have not previously encountered.

When you enter practice, you will encounter many new and different situations. Using the clinical judgment competencies of the Caputi Clinical Judgment Framework provides the support you need as you deal with unfamiliar situations. This support contributes to the development of resiliency and resiliency is a major factor in satisfaction with your work and satisfaction derived from caring for patients. The mental well-being of nurses can be challenging at times, and resiliency supported by a process to think through new challenges supports mental well-being.

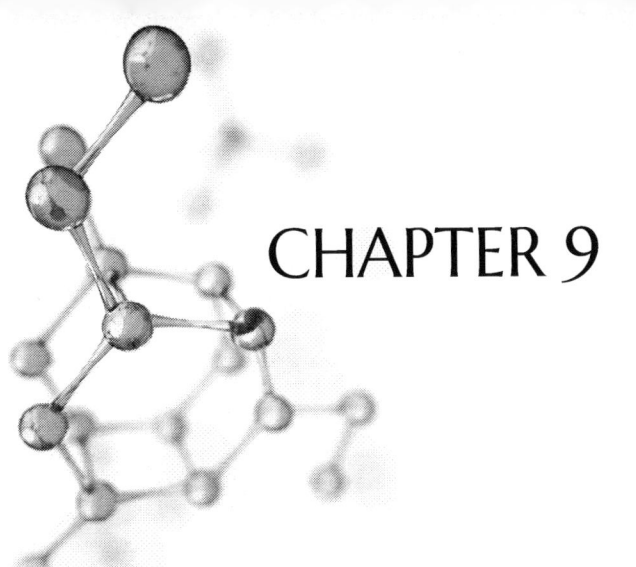

CHAPTER 9

Clinical Judgment Applied to the Healthcare Setting and Care in the Community

AS MENTIONED THROUGHOUT THIS BOOK, clinical judgment is applied to two major aspects of nursing practice. The first is engaging in direct patient care. The second is dealing with issues and problems in the healthcare setting. The nurse is responsible for ensuring a safe healthcare environment that promotes and supports patient safety leading to improved patient outcomes.

The activities in Chapters 3 through 8 focus on thinking used when providing patient care. Chapter 9 provides activities that focus on:

1. Thinking applied to the healthcare setting
2. Care in the community

This chapter provides activities that directly address these two applications of clinical judgment. The nurse must be acutely aware of issues that arise in the healthcare setting and be prepared to deal with those issues to improve the quality of care, the quality of the healthcare environment, and the quality of the overall system. This is a major focus of healthcare known as **quality improvement**. Nurses not only engage in nursing; they also improve nursing. Improving the healthcare setting is a major factor in improving nursing. Again, the overall goal is to improve patient outcomes.

This chapter also includes several activities that address the care of the patient in the **community**. Most nurses begin their career in the acute care or long-term care setting. However, patient care is provided in a variety of settings including in the community. The community itself can be considered a "patient." The community as patient is the focus of public health nursing. The nurse must be able to use clinical judgment in any setting; therefore, this chapter also includes additional thinking activities applied to non-acute care settings.

QUALITY IMPROVEMENT ACTIVITY

MEDICATION ADMINISTRATION FROM A SYSTEMS PERSPECTIVE

Unfortunately, a large number of errors are made that involve medication administration. As previously mentioned, medication administration includes more than the actual delivery of the medication to the patient. This Advanced Level Cognitive Guidance Tool looks at medication administration from a systems perspective. Complete the following tool.

- Accompany a nurse for the day, watching and noting **every** step of the system in which medications are administered—from the time the medication prescription is written until the effects of that medication have been evaluated. Note important aspects of the process then develop a description of the system used in the healthcare agency.

- Identify the top five errors related to medication administration in the healthcare system in which you are working.

Consider the following questions:

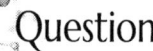Question

What is the overall process to ensure safe administration of medications?

~ How does it work—what are the steps from prescribing to evaluating the effects of the medication?

~ What steps along the way might lead to errors?

~ How can the nurse prevent errors?

~ Were errors made?

~ What happens in that institution when an error is made?

- Go to the "Institute for Safe Medication Practices" website: ismp.org. Identify three areas of this website that can be used to enhance safety when administering medications.

Explaining Your Use of the Clinical Judgment Competencies

What clinical judgment competencies did you use? Complete Table 9.3 at the end of this chapter explaining which clinical judgment competencies you used and how you used each one to complete the activity.

QUALITY IMPROVEMENT ACTIVITY

IMPLEMENTING SAFETY POLICIES

This activity analyzes the safety policies on a nursing care unit and how they are implemented. Review the safety policies in effect on the unit you are working. Example safety policies might include ones related to the use of restraints, falls, and infection control.

Select three policies related to patient safety.
Using Table 9.1 identify three major themes for each policy,
then complete the observations following the table.

TABLE 9.1

Safety Policies

Policy Related to Patient Safety	Major Themes of that Policy
	1
	2
	3
	1
	2
	3
	1
	2
	3

Observe nursing care on the unit.

Based on your observations, cite at least three examples of nursing staff **implementing** each of these policies.

Policy #1:

Policy #2:

Policy #3:

Based on your observations, cite at least three examples of nursing staff **not implementing** each of these policies.

Policy #1:

Policy #2:

Policy #3:

Answer the following questions:

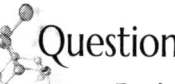Question

Explain why some of the policies were not being implemented as written.

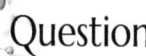Question

What issues or problems may result from not adhering to each of these three policies?

Explaining Your Use of the Clinical Judgment Competencies

What clinical judgment competencies did you use? Complete Table 9.3 at the end of this chapter explaining which clinical judgment competencies you used and how you used each one to complete the activity.

QUALITY IMPROVEMENT ACTIVITY

NATIONAL PATIENT SAFETY GOALS APPLIED TO A COMMUNITY SETTING

In Chapter 8, you used an activity that addressed the National Patient Safety Goals (NPSGs) for a particular clinical area. Review the NPSGs. For each NPSG, discuss how you might apply those same goals when caring for a patient in a community setting.

Identify the type of setting then answer the following questions:

Question
What precautions should the nurse take relative to each safety goal for the patient in the community setting you selected?

Question
Is there a safety goal that is the most important for patients in the community setting you selected?

Question
What information about these patients is most important to communicate to other healthcare providers?

Question

What factors about the environment indicate these safety goals are being met?

Question

What factors about the environment indicate a need for change so the safety goals can be met?

Question

Compare and contrast the implementation of the NPSGs on an inpatient unit with the implementation of the NPSGs in a community setting.

Explaining Your Use of the Clinical Judgment Competencies

What clinical judgment competencies did you use? Complete Table 9.3 at the end of this chapter explaining which clinical judgment competencies you used and how you used each one to complete the activity.

QUALITY IMPROVEMENT ACTIVITY

CONFLICT RESOLUTION

Conflicts are inevitable, especially in a busy, unpredictable healthcare environment. You cannot avoid conflicts in the healthcare setting. The nurse must be skilled at resolving conflict. This activity focuses on an awareness of conflict resolution in the healthcare setting.

- Identify a conflict you observed in the healthcare setting. Describe the conflict, the nature of the issue, and who is involved.

- Observe the interactions of all healthcare professionals in the setting that contributed to the conflict.

Question
How was the conflict actually handled?

- Plan ways you would handle the conflict you identified.

- Compare the way you planned to handle the conflict with the way the conflict was actually handled.

Question
Which approach to handling the conflict was better—the way you planned or the way the conflict was actually handled? Explain.

Explaining Your Use of the Clinical Judgment Competencies

What clinical judgment competencies did you use? Complete Table 9.3 at the end of this chapter explaining which clinical judgment competencies you used and how you used each one to complete the activity.

QUALITY IMPROVEMENT ACTIVITY

ANALYZING THE ELECTRONIC MEDICAL RECORD

Information technology is a major focus in today's healthcare settings. The electronic medical record is convenient to use. Many aspects of these systems are used to ensure safe patient care. The nurse must determine if the systems are properly implemented to ensure safety, must identify any breakdowns, or determine if nurses are using "work arounds" to save time. Work arounds are short cuts that bypass some features that are deemed time consuming. These work arounds often negate the safety aspects of these systems.

Examine an electronic medical record system in a healthcare setting. Answer the following questions:

- Describe the electronic medical record used on the unit. How does its use contribute to safe nursing care?

- Discuss how any data missing on the admission database and/or inconsistencies in documentation affect the accuracy of the information being used to make clinical decisions in the healthcare setting. Was there any information missing in the electronic record and how did that effect safe nursing practice?

- Discuss the benefits of having access to advanced technology in the healthcare setting, such as an electronic medical record and computerized order entry. Note specific advantages of the system you are analyzing.

- What is the nurse's obligation and accountability for ensuring proper documentation of patient data in the electronic medical record?

Explaining Your Use of the Clinical Judgment Competencies

What clinical judgment competencies did you use? Complete Table 9.3 at the end of this chapter explaining which clinical judgment competencies you used and how you used each one to complete the activity.

QUALITY IMPROVEMENT ACTIVITY

CREATING A CULTURE OF SAFETY

Nurses are responsible for the safety of patients. Safety refers to both physical and emotional safety. Establishing a culture of safety provides an environment that is most conducive to the desired patient outcomes. This Advanced Level Cognitive Guidance Tool focuses on safety.

Complete the following information about your patient.

- Age
- Language
- Language barriers
- Physical strength
- Physical limitations
- Cognitive ability (can the patient understand instructions, read signs, understand what the signs mean, etc.)
- Effects the patient's condition may have on safety; explain
- Effects of medications on safety specific for this patient; explain
- Environment
- Tubes
- Equipment
- Assistance available to help the patient
- Identification band on?
- Allergy band on?
- Current information on the patient board
- Call light available
- Add any further information or precautions you identified that are specific for this patient

The nurse considers all the above information and uses it to plan interventions to keep the patient safe.

*Based on the above information you collected,
use Table 9.2 to list the information that indicates a potential safety issue
for this patient and plan interventions to ensure safety.*

TABLE 9.2

Identifying Safety Issues

Factors indicating a safety issue	Factors about the care unit that present risks for this patient	Interventions to prevent harm from the identified safety issue

Add additional rows as needed

Explaining Your Use of the Clinical Judgment Competencies

What clinical judgment competencies did you use? Complete Table 9.3 at the end of this chapter explaining which clinical judgment competencies you used and how you used each one to complete the activity.

COMMUNITY ACTIVITY

COMMUNITY ASSESSMENT/WINDSHIELD SURVEY

Just as you assess a patient, you assess a community. This tool guides you through a community assessment. Many clinical judgment competencies are used in the collection of this data and the analysis of the data to determine community needs.

To complete this activity, you will conduct a community assessment by driving through a neighborhood and collecting data based on what you are seeing through the "windshield" of your car.

Boundaries

- Are there geographic or physical boundaries such as a highway, railroad, lake, river, a different terrain, presence of industrial or commercial units along with residential?
- Does the neighborhood have an identity, a name? If so, is it displayed?
- Does the neighborhood have an unofficial name?
- Are there sub-communities within the area?

Housing and Zoning

- How old are the houses? What is the style of houses and what types of materials were used in their construction?
- Are all the neighborhood houses similar?
- If not, how would you characterize the differences?
- Are there single or multi-family homes or both?
- What size are the lots (approximately)?
- Are there signs of disrepair such as broken doors, steps, windows, and unkempt yards?
- Are there vacant houses?
- Does the neighborhood show signs of improvements or signs of decay?
- Is it "alive?" How would you decide?
- Is there trash, abandoned cars, boarded up buildings, rubble, dilapidated buildings, and cluttered vacant lots?
- Is there evidence of poor drainage, potential disease, and breeding places for disease-producing organisms to grow?

Parks and Recreational Areas

- Are there parks and recreational areas in the neighborhood? Are there green spaces?
- Is the open space public or private?
- Who uses these spaces?

Common Areas

- Are there areas where people congregate? Describe those areas.
- What groups of people congregate and at what hours?
- Do these gathering areas have a sense of territoriality or are they open to strangers?

Stores

- What supermarkets or neighborhood stores are available?
- How do residents travel to the store?
- Are there drug stores, laundries, dry cleaners, and other services in the area?

Transportation

- How do people get in and out of the neighborhood?
- What is the condition of the streets?
- Is there a major highway near the neighborhood?
- Is public transportation available and is that public transportation available to all in the area such as the elderly and disabled?

Service Centers

- Are there social agencies, recreation centers, schools, and libraries?
- Are there healthcare providers such as physicians, dentists, clinics, emergency departments, hospitals, and long-term care facilities?

People on the Street

- Who is on the street—women, children, teenagers, community health nurses, collection agents, salespeople?
- How are they dressed?
- What animals do you see, such as strays, pets, other?

Protective Services
- Is there evidence of police in the area?
- Is there evidence of fire protection in the area?

Race
- Are there various racial groups in the neighborhood? If so, what racial groups are represented?
- How many different groups?

Ethnicity and Religion
- What churches and church schools are in the neighborhood?
- How many are there?

Socioeconomic Level
- How would you categorize socioeconomic level of the residents?
- On what do you base your decisions?

Health and Safety
- Is there evidence of potential accidents, substance abuse, poor lighting on streets, poor sidewalk/street conditions? On what do you base this judgment?
- Are cyclists wearing helmets?
- Are sidewalks clear of snow/ice (in winter), other obstacles?

Summary of Your Overall Assessment of the Community
- What is your impression of this community?
- Conduct an internet search of the community. What are the major health concerns for this area? What are the crime statistics for the community?
- Describe the populations in the community that are the most vulnerable and at risk for access to health care.

Explaining Your Use of the Clinical Judgment Competencies

What clinical judgment competencies did you use? Complete Table 9.3 at the end of this chapter explaining which clinical judgment competencies you used and how you used each one to complete the activity.

TABLE 9.3

Explaining Your Thinking Using the Caputi Clinical Judgment Framework

Name of Activity:_____

Clinical Judgment Competencies	Which Clinical Judgment Competency Was Used and How it Was Used
Getting the Information 1. Determining important information to collect 2. Scanning the environment 3. Identifying signs and symptoms 4. Assessing systematically and comprehensively 5. Ensuring accurate information	
Making Meaning of the Information 1. Clustering related information 2. Identifying assumptions 3. Recognizing inconsistencies 4. Distinguishing relevant from irrelevant information 5. Judging how much ambiguity is acceptable 6. Comparing and contrasting 7. Predicting potential complications 8. Collaborating with healthcare team members 9. Determining patient care needs/healthcare environment issues	

TABLE 9.3 (continued)

Explaining Your Thinking Using the Caputi Clinical Judgment Framework

Clinical Judgment Competencies	Which Clinical Judgment Competency Was Used and How it Was Used
Determining Actions to Take 1. Selecting interventions 2. Managing potential complications 3. Setting priorities	
Taking Action 1. Determining how to implement the planned interventions 2. Delegating (Assigning for some PN/VNs) 3. Communicating 4. Teaching others	
Evaluating Outcomes and Your Thinking 1. Evaluating data 2. Evaluating and correcting thinking	

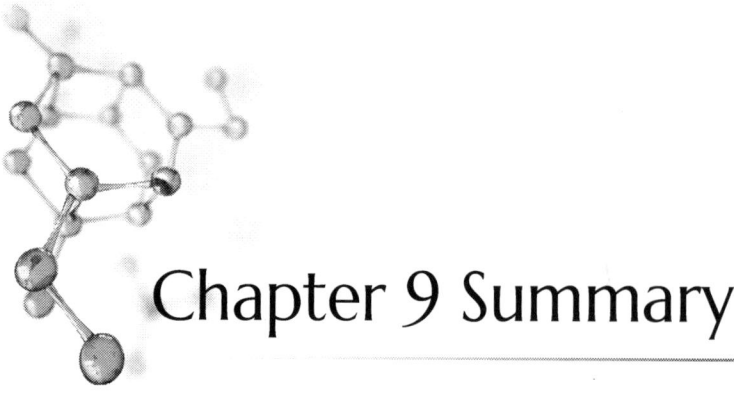

Chapter 9 Summary

Chapter 9's Advanced Level Cognitive Guidance Tools expand your thinking by requiring you to use many clinical judgment competencies with one activity. These activities focused on the clinical environment and care in the community. The Caputi Clinical Judgment Framework is a flexible framework that can be used to make all types of decisions in the healthcare environment.

Using the tools in Chapter 9, you once again explained your thinking in both terms of content and clinical judgment competencies. The goal of this practice is for you to learn that only using content to explain your thinking does not actually explain your thinking. Reflecting on your thinking to deal with issues that may arise in the healthcare environment increases your awareness of real-world nursing. Although the bulk of your nursing education is focused on patient care, a good deal of time in the nurse's day is dedicated to dealing with issues in the healthcare environment to ensure all aspects of patient care are safe.

Additionally, nurses work in many positions other than providing direct patient care. Examples of these non-direct patient care positions include unit manager, charge nurse, and healthcare advocate with public health departments. All areas of nursing require the nurse to engage in sound problem-solving and decision making. That thinking is best accomplished implementing clinical judgment using the Caputi Clinical Judgment Framework.

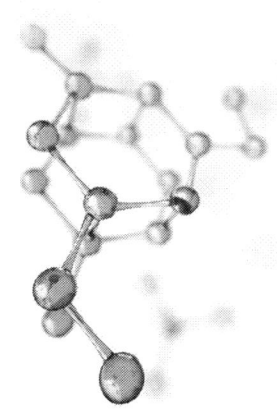 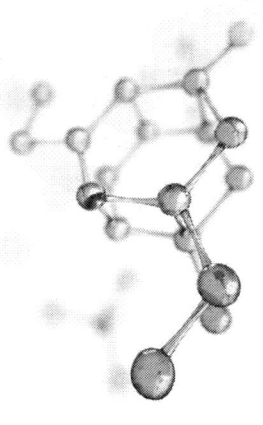

SECTION III

Controlling Your Own Thinking: Becoming a Self-Directed Thinker by Using the Caputi Clinical Judgment Framework

(Chapter 10)

SECTION III OF THIS BOOK has just one chapter. The purpose of this chapter is to pull together all that you learned in this book and provide ideas on how to use all the clinical judgment competencies of the Caputi Clinical Judgment Framework. The activities are designed to guide you as a self-directed thinker. As discussed in Chapter 1, one reason for learning the Caputi Clinical Judgment Framework is to become a self-directed thinker. You learned all the pieces of the framework in Section I of this book. Then in Section II you applied the thinking of the framework to many thinking activities then explained how you used the various clinical judgment competencies.

Section III reveals ideas about how to bring all that information together and apply the framework in various learning environments. Chapter 10, Putting it All Together, presents an example of how a student used Step 1 of the Caputi Clinical Judgment Framework to explain her thinking and provides ways to use the framework while learning throughout the nursing program. The chapter then turns to using the Caputi Clinical Judgment Framework after graduation. During interviews with nurse recruiters, you may be asked to explain how you solve problems and make decisions as a nurse. You can discuss your knowledge of the Caputi Clinical Judgment Framework and explain how you used it to think like a nurse throughout your nursing program. Additionally, in your first nursing position you can ask your preceptor for feedback about your thinking in terms of the clinical judgment competencies of the framework.

Section III helps you "pull it all together" to become a self-directed thinker in school and in your professional practice. And best of all, the Caputi Clinical Judgment Framework can be used in any nursing area of practice so you can use it wherever your career takes you.

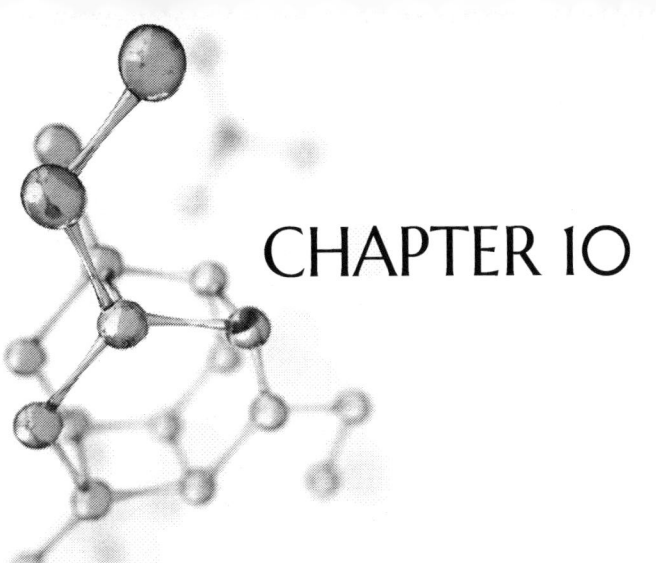

CHAPTER 10

Putting It All Together

AS DISCUSSED IN CHAPTER 1 of this book, there are many reasons for learning about clinical judgment and how to use clinical judgment in nursing. These reasons include:

1. Preparing for the NCLEX

2. Transforming your everyday thinking to clinical judgment for safe patient care and to improve patient outcomes

3. Becoming resilient

4. Becoming a self-directed thinker

5. Using situation-based thinking

6. Dealing with unexpected occurrences and reducing errors in the healthcare setting

Of the six items on the list, number 4, "becoming a self-directed thinker," is the end goal. Your faculty will ask you many questions in the classroom, in simulation, and especially in the clinical setting. You must be prepared to **not** just provide content answers (which labs to look at; what medications the patient is on), but you must also explain the thinking you used to determine that you must look at the lab results or the medications prescribed. As you learn how to think, your clinical judgment thinking will become more automatic. With enough practice using all the clinical judgment competencies taught in Chapters 3 through 7, your thinking should become so automatic that you will find yourself using the clinical judgment competencies to actually direct your thinking. When you reach that point, you are a self-directed thinker.

When reaching the goal of becoming a self-directed thinker, you will be better prepared for each of the following:

1. The NCLEX
2. Being resilient
3. Using situation-based thinking
4. Unexpected occurrences and reducing errors in the healthcare setting

What does a self-directed thinker using the Caputi Clinical Judgment Framework look like? Let's look at an example. This example is the report from a self-directed thinking student in the final semester of a nursing program. The student reports on using Step 1 of the Caputi Clinical Framework: "Getting the Information."

CAPUTI CLINICAL JUDGMENT FRAMEWORK

Step 1: Getting the Information
Determining Important Information to Collect

Below is the information I received from the previous nurse's report, and the important information I will collect based on that report.

- During report from the nurse on the previous shift and from a review of the SBAR report, I learned the patient was admitted with pneumonia. Information to collect: a complete respiratory assessment including lung sounds, laboratory tests such as sputum culture results, medications the patient is taking to treat the pneumonia, and the complete blood count results taken three hours earlier with comparison to previous readings, especially the white blood cell count.

- The patient was reported to be oriented X4 throughout the previous shift. I will assess level of consciousness and orientation.

- Pulse oximetry reported to have been between 90 and 92: measure pulse ox with initial assessment.

- The nurse stated the patient was watching TV during most of previous shift, but states is growing tired; frequent yawning: I will assess the patient's readiness for sleep.

CAPUTI CLINICAL JUDGMENT FRAMEWORK

Step 1: Getting the Information
Scanning the Environment

Upon entering the room, I noted an IV infusing on an infusion pump; "fall risk" written on the communication board in the room noting ambulation with x1 assist; oxygen cannula incorrectly placed, tubing hanging around the patient's neck; and the oxygen flow rate set at 2 liters. There was a food tray from dinner that was delivered two hours ago with about half of the meal still on the tray. There was one visitor at the bedside.

CAPUTI CLINICAL JUDGMENT FRAMEWORK

Step 1: Getting the Information
Identifying Signs and Symptoms

During my initial assessment I noted the patient's facial skin color was pale and slightly bluish around the mouth; appeared to be sleeping; difficulty arousing, only aroused with tactile stimuli. The visitor stated the patient has been sleeping for the last 15 minutes.

CAPUTI CLINICAL JUDGMENT FRAMEWORK

Step 1: Getting the Information
Assessing Systematically & Comprehensively

With the unexpected finding of facial skin color and difficulty arousing, I applied my knowledge of perfusion to consider all assessment data to collect (a deeper, focused assessment) and what immediate actions that may need to be taken related to decreased perfusion. I collected the following information and immediately implemented a couple interventions:

- Color of nail beds; capillary refill; skin temperature

- Pulse oximetry reading, blood pressure, pulse

- No dyspnea or edema

- Lung sounds; respiratory rate and character

- Repositioned oxygen cannula and ensured oxygen was set at correct flow rate

- Positioned patient for lung expansion

- Assessed the patient's level of consciousness: awakens to tactile stimuli only; oriented X4 but slow to respond; reports feeling dizzy; denies chest discomfort

- Asked the patient "how are things going for you today?" and "tell me about this dizziness you are having."

- Reviewed medical record for last 24 hours, reading the nurse's notes and notes from the respiratory therapist and primary care provider

- Reviewed medication administration record for any medications that may have an effect on the patient's state of perfusion

CAPUTI CLINICAL JUDGMENT FRAMEWORK

Step I: Getting the Information
Ensuring Accurate Information

I needed to ensure the information I collected was accurate. Accurate data collection first starts with my level of knowledge of perfusion, related pathophysiology, and the individual patient situation. I must be fully informed. Following is how I determined the accuracy of the data I collected or how I will determine the accuracy should I doubt what I am collecting:

- Pulse ox: If unsure the equipment is working correctly, I will take my own pulse ox to test the device.

- Lung sounds: If I am in doubt about what I am hearing, I will consult with another nurse to assess.

- Ensure oxygen is flowing: Check for correct flow rate set on the flow meter; ensure the oxygen cannula is placed correctly; check for kinks in the tubing.

- Determine patient's ability to provide reliable information: Review medical record for any evidence of the patient's inability to be a reliable historian. Check the accuracy of the patient's response to questions related to orientation.

This student's report demonstrates the use of the Caputi Clinical Judgment Framework when "Getting the Information." In so doing, the student demonstrated thinking that was patient-centered and situation-based. It provides a foundation for resiliency because the student has a process to follow for mindful thinking, ensuring attention is centered on the patient.

Finally, using the Caputi Clinical Judgment Framework helps the student deal with unexpected occurrences, focusing on the patient's needs and nursing actions to reduce errors in patient care. The student would then address the next four steps of the Caputi Clinical Judgment Framework, explaining how each of the clinical judgment competencies was used. This approach develops a self-directed thinker. As is evidenced by the student's report, the necessary, important **content** about the patient is determined by applying thinking.

Using the Caputi Clinical Judgment Framework to Become a Self-Directed Thinker Throughout Your Nursing Program

There are several ways to use the Caputi Clinical Judgment Framework to become a self-directed thinker during your nursing program. Most important is to have the entire framework readily available. Print a copy of the Caputi Clinical Judgment Framework with the five steps and the 23 related clinical judgment competencies. Shrink that page into the size of a notecard, then laminate the page to make it a card you can easily wipe clean. Take that card with you to your classroom sessions, simulation lab experiences, and clinical setting. Use that card to direct your thinking.

A Study and Care Planning Tool

Using the Complete Caputi Clinical Judgment Framework as a Study and Care Planning Tool

There are many ways to use the Caputi Clinical Judgment Framework to learn nursing. Consider the entire framework as presented in Table 10.1.

TABLE 10.1

The Caputi Clinical Judgment Framework

Name of Activity:_____

Clinical Judgment Competencies	Which Clinical Judgment Competency Was Used and How it Was Used
Getting the Information 1. Determining important information to collect 2. Scanning the environment 3. Identifying signs and symptoms 4. Assessing systematically and comprehensively 5. Ensuring accurate information	

TABLE 10.1 *(continued)*

The Caputi Clinical Judgment Framework

Clinical Judgment Competencies	Which Clinical Judgment Competency Was Used and How it Was Used
Making Meaning of the Information 1. Clustering related information 2. Identifying assumptions 3. Recognizing inconsistencies 4. Distinguishing relevant from irrelevant information 5. Judging how much ambiguity is acceptable 6. Comparing and contrasting 7. Predicting potential complications 8. Collaborating with healthcare team members 9. Determining patient care needs/healthcare environment issues	
Determining Actions to Take 1. Selecting interventions 2. Managing potential complications 3. Setting priorities	
Taking Action 1. Determining how to implement the planned interventions 2. Delegating (Assigning for some PN/VNs) 3. Communicating 4. Teaching others	
Evaluating Outcomes and Your Thinking 1. Evaluating data 2. Evaluating and correcting thinking	

This chapter provides ideas about how to use the information in the table to help you study nursing content, plan patient care, discuss your thinking in simulation debriefing, and explain your thinking in the clinical setting.

Study Pathophysiology and Learn about Medications

Using the Complete Caputi Clinical Judgment Framework to Study Pathophysiology and Learn about Medications

Consider using the Caputi Clinical Judgment Framework as you learn pathophysiology. The importance of learning pathophysiology is to know how to relate the pathology content to the care of the patient. Not all, but many of the clinical judgment competencies are needed to frame your thinking when planning patient care based on the pathophysiology of a medical diagnosis. You might apply some of the competencies to learn about, or organize your thoughts about, the pathology. You can then complete the framework when you are caring for a patient with that pathology.

For example, to first organize your clinical judgment when learning about the pathology of pneumonia, you might consider entering the information as noted with italics in Table 10.2. The clinical judgment competencies to address **while learning about the pathology are bolded**. The information obtained about the pathology when applying the bolded clinical judgment competencies will be used when you apply the remaining clinical judgment competencies when caring for a patient with that medical diagnosis. Table 10.2 provides an example using the pathology of pneumonia.

TABLE 10.2

Organizing Your Learning about Pneumonia

The Pathophysiology of Pneumonia: Lungs are congested with fluid; airways are narrowed.

Clinical Judgment Competencies	Which Clinical Judgment Competency Was Used and How it Was Used
1. GETTING THE INFORMATION	
Determining important information to collect	*What information will you collect from the medical record?*
Scanning the environment	*What do you expect to be in the room of a patient diagnosed with this pathophysiology?*
Identifying signs and symptoms	*What signs and symptoms will you assess for patients in an acute care setting with this pathophysiology?*
Assessing systematically and comprehensively	*What additional data will you collect for specific groups of patients with this pathology, such as—if the patient was pregnant, elderly, or a child? Or for patients with other pre-existing conditions?*
Ensuring accurate information	

TABLE 10.2 *(continued)*

Organizing Your Learning about Pneumonia

Clinical Judgment Competencies	Which Clinical Judgment Competency Was Used and How it Was Used
2. MAKING MEANING OF THE INFORMATION	
Clustering related information	*Which signs and symptoms can you cluster together that might point to a particular patient care issue? Example: low pulse ox and wheezing may result in difficulty ambulating.*
Identifying assumptions	
Recognizing inconsistencies	*Are there any inconsistencies between what you learned about this pathology and what the patient is actually displaying?*
Distinguishing relevant from irrelevant information	
Judging how much ambiguity is acceptable	*What are the changes in patient information (such as vital signs, laboratory data, limitations with ADLs) that are expected and at what point would those changes be unacceptable and require intervention? For example, a patient with bacterial pneumonia will have a fever, but at what point would the fever be too high and what should the nurse do if that occurs?*
Comparing and contrasting	
Predicting potential complications	*What complications may result if the manifestations of the pathology are not addressed?*
Collaborating with healthcare team members	*What other healthcare team members would be involved in the care of a patient with this pathology?*
Determining patient care needs/healthcare environment issues	

TABLE 10.2 *(continued)*

Organizing Your Learning about Pneumonia

3. DETERMINING ACTIONS TO TAKE	
Selecting interventions	What are the typical nursing interventions and medical interventions for this pathology?
Managing potential complications	For the potential complications you identified above, how will you prevent them from happening? What will you do if they happen?
Setting priorities	For this pathology, what are the primary assessments to make?
4. TAKING ACTION	
Determining how to implement the planned interventions	
Assigning and Delegating	
Communicating	What information will you include on the SBAR report for the oncoming nurse?
Teaching others	What is important information to teach a patient with this pathology?
5. EVALUATING OUTCOMES AND YOUR THINKING	
Evaluating data	
Evaluating and correcting thinking	

Using the above approach consistently while learning pathophysiology provides a systematic process for your learning. It demonstrates how what you are learning about pathophysiology will actually be used when caring for patients.

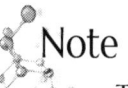

Note

The above-described approach for learning pathophysiology can also be applied to learn about medications. Completing the table with each pathology you learn and for each medication you learn gives you the basic information that you will use and the thinking you will apply to plan patient care. Completing these tables also provides an excellent approach for organizing what you are learning when studying for the NCLEX. Keep these and use these completed tables when studying for NCLEX to focus on both content and thinking!

Using the Complete Caputi Clinical Judgment Framework in the Clinical Setting

In the Clinical Setting

In the **final term** (semester, quarter, or other system your school uses) you should approach patient care guided by your own thinking. You have learned the entire framework and all the clinical judgment competencies. You have practiced applying individual competencies as well as explaining how you used those competencies when working through clinical judgment activities. Now is the time for you to use the framework to guide your thinking.

After you receive information about your patient from the nurse or your faculty, begin to fill in Table 10.1 with the information you received. During your initial visit with your patient, continue to fill in the table with other information you collect, as guided by applying the clinical judgment competencies under Step 1: "Getting the Information." At this point you are likely collecting and processing patient information automatically, having had practice using this approach.

Once you have filled in all the information to collect, review the table to determine if there is anything you are missing. Finally, complete Step 2: "Making Meaning of the Information" and Step 3: "Determining Actions to Take." Use these steps to guide you through the day. You may at times need to return to prior clinical judgment competencies to update the patient information and your thinking as your patient's condition changes. Throughout the day you will also complete Step 4: "Taking Action" and Step 5: "Evaluating Outcomes and Your Thinking."

You can also use the framework during post-conference discussions when explaining the decisions you made and how you made them. Keep implementing this approach to patient care throughout the term to reach the end goal of becoming a self-directed thinker.

Keep in mind that as you work through the Caputi Clinical Judgment Framework you are implementing the nursing process. Refer to Table 10.3 first presented in Chapter 2.

TABLE 10.3

Alignment of the NCSBN Clinical Judgment Measurement Model, the Caputi Clinical Judgment Framework, and the Steps of the Nursing Process

The Cognitive Processes of the NCSBN Clinical Judgment Measurement Model (Next Generation NCLEX)	Major Steps in the Caputi Clinical Judgment Framework	Steps of the Nursing Process
1. Recognize Cues	Getting the Information	Assessing
2. Analyze Cues	Making Meaning of the Information	Diagnosing
3. Prioritize Hypotheses	Determining Actions to Take	Planning
4. Generate Solutions	Determining Actions to Take	Planning
5. Take Actions	Taking Action	Implementing
6. Evaluate Outcomes	Evaluating Outcomes and Your Thinking	Evaluating

As demonstrated with this table, when implementing the Caputi Clinical Judgment Framework you are implementing all steps of the nursing process and learning the cognitive processes that are tested on the NCLEX.

Using the Complete Caputi Clinical Judgment Framework in Simulation

Because the high-fidelity simulation experience simulates real-world nursing practice, clinical judgment is incorporated as a vital part of your learning. Simulation is often touted to be a primary learning activity for teaching students to think like a nurse. However, meeting the goal of thinking like a nurse must be intentional and deliberate. Working through a simulation experience requires the application of an organized approach to thinking and the Caputi Clinical Judgment Framework can be used for this purpose.

If faculty provide information about the patient scenario prior to the start of the simulation, begin filling in Table 10.1 to organize your thinking. Consider which clinical judgment competencies will be most important for you to use in the simulation. Use those clinical judgment competencies to guide your thinking.

During post-simulation debriefing, use Table 10.1 to guide your thinking. If you laminated a pocket-sized card with the Caputi Clinical Judgment Framework on it, pull it out. Use it to discuss the thinking you used and the decisions you made. This is a perfect way to demonstrate that you are reaching the goal of thinking like a nurse by explaining your thinking using the words and language of the Clinical Judgment Framework. The language of the clinical judgment competencies helps you bring content and clinical judgment together—you use clinical judgment language to talk about how you used the patient information of the scenario to make decisions. Now you are thinking like a nurse!

In Simulation

Using the Complete Caputi Clinical Judgment Framework to Work Through Case Studies in the Classroom

Print out a table for each of the five steps of the Caputi Clinical Judgment Framework on a separate sheet of paper. Make the table big enough to add information. As your faculty works through a case study in the classroom, insert on the table the information discussed. Table 10.4 presents an example of what you might include in a table addressing Step 1 of the Caputi Clinical Judgment Framework: "Getting the Information."

In the Classroom

TABLE 10.4

Applying Clinical Judgment Competencies to Case Studies

TOPIC: (insert here information that identifies the type of case study)

Clinical Judgment Competency	Notes Related to the Clinical Judgment Competency
GETTING THE INFORMATION	
Determining Important Information to Collect	What information in the case study leads to specific information you should collect?
Scanning the Environment	Consider the environment of the patient in the case study. What is that specific environment (home health, clinic, in-patient acute care, long-term care)? What should you look for? What does the case study tell you about the healthcare environment?
Identifying Signs and Symptoms	Basic pathophysiology related to the patient's condition and assessment data to collect.
Assessing Systematically and Comprehensively	Additional information to collect related to the assessment data provided: perhaps reviewing meds, labs; patient's history; other healthcare provider information—what would you be looking for?
Ensuring Accurate Information	How do you know the patient is an accurate historian? Is there any information you should question?

Continue with another page for each of the remaining four steps of the framework.

Your First Nursing Position Interview

You might be asking why your first nursing position interview is a topic for this chapter. A common concern of nurse managers is that newly graduated nurses are not able to engage in quality decision-making.

Prior to 2023 the NCLEX did not actually test clinical judgment. The National Council of State Boards of Nursing's research confirmed the NCLEX did not test the level of clinical judgment needed by new nurse graduates. For that reason, the NCLEX changed starting in 2023 and was titled the Next Generation NCLEX because it represented a major change and began measuring a much higher level of thinking. However, keep in mind that even with the Next Generation NCLEX, the NCLEX only measures **minimal competency** of newly graduated nurses. The goal of all nursing programs is to teach students how to engage in good clinical judgment so their decisions are high quality and not just those needed for **minimal competency**.

During your interview the nurse recruiter will ask many questions. They typically want to know what kinds of experiences you had during nursing school. Some may ask you how you approach a problem. Of course, you will answer that you use the nursing process, **BUT** you should definitely share what you learned about clinical judgment as the thinking behind the nursing process and how you used clinical judgment to make good decisions.

Explain to the nurse recruiter the Caputi Clinical Judgment Framework and all the clinical judgment competencies you learned. Talk about how you used this framework to approach patient care and solve other problems in the healthcare environment. You may want to share that having this framework kept you focused and mindful about how to care for your patient from a patient-centered perspective.

When you are working in your first nursing position, an experienced nurse will serve as a preceptor and guide on what is expected on the unit where you are working. A common problem preceptors experience is trying to guide new graduates in making good decisions. It would be extremely helpful for you to share the Caputi Clinical Judgment Framework with your preceptor and explain how you learned to think using the framework. You might ask your preceptor to help you grow in your thinking by giving you feedback on your thinking using the language of the framework. This will be very helpful to you, but also very helpful for your preceptor, who will likely appreciate having a language to use to provide feedback on your thinking.

Definitely share what you learned about clinical judgment as the thinking behind the nursing process and how you used clinical judgment to make good decisions in your nursing interviews.

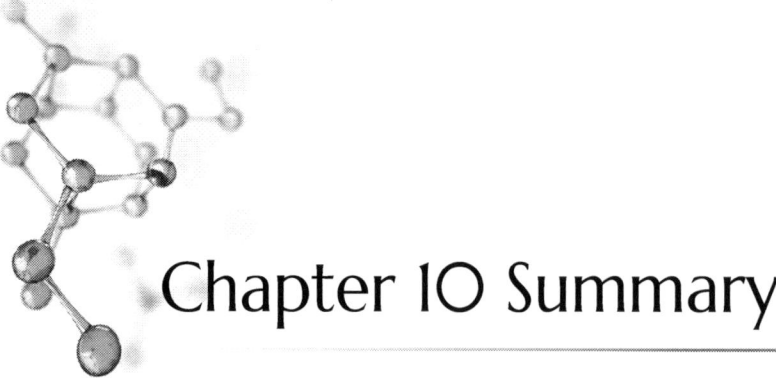

Chapter 10 Summary

Chapter 10 is titled "Putting it All Together" because the end goal is for the student to pull together everything learned about the Caputi Clinical Judgment Framework as an approach to solving problems and making good care decisions in nursing. The total framework is used to guide thinking, provide confidence in approaching decisions, support resiliency, ensure patient-centered nursing, and result in good decisions made throughout nursing school and in the future by reflecting on and correcting thinking.

Thank you for taking the Caputi Clinical Judgment Framework with you on your journey to becoming a nurse. I wish you the best in your nursing career.

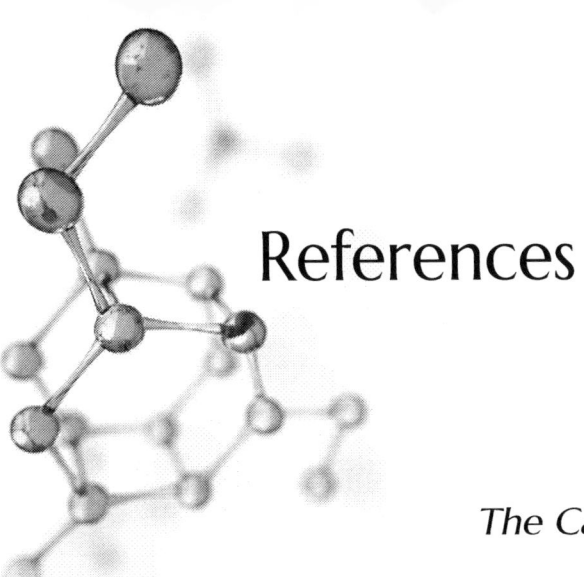

References

Think Like a Nurse
The Caputi Method for Learning Clinical Judgment

Andel, C., Davidow, S. L., Holland, M., & Moreno, D. A. (2012). The economics of healthcare quality and medical errors, *Journal of Health Care Finance*, 39(1), 39-50.

**Benner, P. (2001). *From novice to expert: Excellence and power in clinical nursing practice.* (Commemorative Edition). Prentice Hall.

Brown, P. C., Roediger, H. L., & McDaniel, M. A. (2014). *Make it stick.* Belknap Press of Harvard University Press.

Burton, M. A., Smith, D. W., & Ludwig, L. J. (2019). *Fundamentals of nursing care: Concepts, connections, & skills,* (3rd ed.), F. A. Davis.

Cannon, S., & Boswell, C. (Eds.) (2016). *Evidence-based teaching in nursing: A foundation for educators,* (2nd ed.), Jones & Bartlett.

Capelletti, A., Engel, J. K., & Prentice, D. (2014). Systematic review of clinical judgment and reasoning in nursing. *Journal of Nursing Education, 53* (8), 453-458. https://doi-org.georgian.idm.oclc.org/10.3928/01484834-20140724-01

Caputi, L. (2010a). An introduction to developing critical thinking in nursing education. In L. Caputi, (Ed.), *Teaching nursing: The art and science* (2nd ed., Vol 2, pp. 381-390). DuPage Press.

Caputi, L. (2010b). Operationalizing critical thinking. In L. Caputi, (Ed.), *Teaching nursing: The art and science* (2nd ed., Vol. 2, pp. 381-390). DuPage Press.

Caputi, L. (2016). The Caputi model for teaching thinking in nursing, in L. Caputi, (Ed.), Innovations in nursing education: Building the future of nursing (2nd ed., Vol. 3, pp. 3-12). Wolters Kluwer.

Caputi, L. (2020). *Think Like a Nurse: A Handbook* (Rev. ed.). Windy City Publishers.

Gélinas, C. (2018). Pain assessment and management. In B. Kozier, G. Erb, A. Berman, S. J. Synder, G Frandsen, M. Buck, L. Ferguson, L. Yiu, & L. L. & Stamler (Eds.), *Fundamentals of Canadian nursing: Concepts, process, and practice* (4th Canadian ed., pp. 668-709). Pearson Canada.

Hanson, R. (2018). *Resilient.* Harmony Book.

Haslam, L. (2019). Pain assessment. In C. Jarvis, A. J. Browne, J. MacDonald-Jenkins, & M. Luctkar-Flude (Eds.), *Jarvis physical examination & health assessment.* (3rd Canadian ed., pp. 182-195). Elsevier Canada.

Institute of Medicine (IOM). (2011). *The future of nursing: Leading change, advancing health.* The National Academies Press.

International Association for the Study of Pain. (n. d.). *IASP terminology: Pain.* IASP. https://www.iasp-pain.org/resources/terminology/#pain

Kavanagh, J. M., & Szweda, C. (2017). A crisis in competency: The strategic and ethical imperative to assessing new graduate nurses' clinical reasoning. *Nursing Education Perspectives, 38,* (2), 57-62.

Koharchik, L., Caputi, L., Robb, M., & Culleiton, A. (2015). Fostering clinical reasoning in nursing students. *American Journal of Nursing, 115,* (1), 58-61.

Lasater, K. (2011). Clinical judgment: The last frontier for evaluation. *Nurse Education in Process, 11,* 86-92.

Makary, M. A., & Daniel, M. (2016). Medical error—the third leading cause of death in the US. *British Medical Journal, 353:* doi: http://dx.doi.org/10.1136/bmj.i2139

Muntean, W. J. (2012). *Nursing clinical decision-making: A literature review.* Paper commissioned by the National Council of State Boards of Nursing.

National Council of State Boards of Nursing (Winter, 2019). *Next Generation NCLEX News, Clinical judgment measurement model,* https://www.ncsbn.org/13342.htm

National Council of State Boards of Nursing & American Nurses Association. (2019). *National guidelines for nursing delegation,* https://www.ncsbn.org/13546.htm

Nielsen, A. & Lasater, K. (2021), Clinical judgment. In J. Giddens, Ed., *Concepts for nursing practice,* (2nd ed., pp. 371-380). Elsevier.

Nilson, L. B. (2013). *Creating self-regulated learners.* Stylus.

Odell, M. (2015). Detection and management of the deteriorating ward patient: An evaluation of nursing practice. *Journal of Clinical Nursing, 24*(1–2), 173. https://doi-org.georgian.idm.oclc.org/10.1111/jocn.12655

Panadero, E., Alonso-Tapia, J., & Reche, E. (2013). Rubrics vs. self-assessment scripts effect on self-regulation, performance, and self-efficacy in pre-service teachers. *Studies in Educational Evaluation, 39,* 125-132.

Paul, R., & Elder, L. (2020). *The miniature guide to critical thinking: Concepts and tools* (8th ed.). Rowman & Littlefield.

Purling, A., & King, L. (2012). A literature review: Graduate nurses' preparedness for recognising and responding to the deteriorating patient. *Journal of Clinical Nursing,* 21, 3451-3465.

Rubenfeld, M. G., & Scheffer, B. K. (2015). *Critical thinking TACTICS for nurses: Achieving the IOM competencies.* (3rd ed.). Jones & Bartlett.

Sawhney, M., & Martelli, B. L. (2019). Pain assessment and management. In P. A. Potter, A. G. Perry, P. A. Stockert, A. M. Hall, B. J. Astle, & W. Duggleby (Eds.), *Canadian fundamentals of nursing* (6th Canadian ed., pp. 575-610). Elsevier Canada.

Sheridan, C. (2016). *The mindful nurse: Using the power of mindfulness and compassion to help you think in your work.* Rivertime Press.

Shinnick, M. A., & Woo, M. A. (2018). Validation of time to task performance assessment method in simulation: A comparative design study. *Nurse Educator Today,* 64, 108-114. DOI:10.1016/j.nedt.2018.02.011.

Sieg, D. (2020). *7 habits of highly resilient nurses,* Sigma Theta Tau Nursing Center. https://nursingcentered.sigmanursing.org/features/more-features/Vol41_1_7-habits-of-highly-resilient-nurses

**Tanner, C. (2006). Thinking like a nurse: A research-based model of clinical judgment in nursing. *Journal of Nursing Education, 45*(6), 204-211.

Tyo, M. B., & McCurry, M. K. (2019). An integrative review of clinical reasoning teaching strategies and outcome evaluation in nursing education, *Nursing Education Perspectives, 40*(1), 11-17.

White, A., Maguire, M. B. R., Brannan, J., & Brown, A. (2021). Situational awareness in acute patient deterioration, *Nurse Educator, 46*(2), 82-86 DOI: 10.1097/NNE.0000000000000968.

**Indicates classic reference.

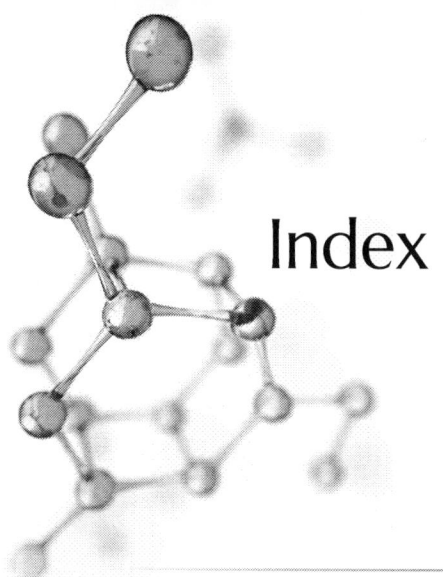

Index

Think Like a Nurse
The Caputi Method for Learning Clinical Judgment

A

ABCD Prioritization Model, 162–165
Advanced Level Cognitive Guidance Tools. See cognitive guidance tools, advanced
adverse events
 dealing with, 18–19
 Managing Potential Complications, 154–158, 226–227, 290
 Predicting Potential Complications, 127–131, 226–227, 290
 Teaching Others and, 186–189, 241–242, 290
ambiguity, 118–122
Analyze Cues, NCLEX Clinical Judgment Measurement Model, 7, 9. *See also* Making Meaning of Information, Caputi Clinical Judgment Framework
applying thinking, 211–213. *See also* cognitive guidance tools, advanced; self-directed thinkers
asking for help, importance of, 32–33
Assessing, nursing process, 45–47
Assessing Systematically and Comprehensively, 74–81
 Caputi Framework for study of pathophysiology and medications, 288–290
 defined, 74
 self-directed thinking, putting it all together, 284
assessment data, 197
assumptions, identifying, 100–105

B

bias
 Identifying Assumptions, 100–105
 preconceived ideas and attitudes, information gathering and, 32–33
bigger picture thinking, 26–27. *See also* Making Meaning of Information
 Clustering Related Information, 94–99
 Judging How Much Ambiguity is Acceptable, 118–122

C

Caputi Clinical Judgment Framework. *See also* main entry for each framework step
 clinical judgment competencies, 41–44
 Determining Actions to Take step, 34–35
 Evaluating Outcomes and Thinking step, 36–37
 Getting the Information step, 31, 32–33
 Learning Activity, 38–41
 Making Meaning of Information step, 33–34
 NCLEX Clinical Judgment Measurement Model and, 8–10, 30
 nursing process and, 45–47
 resilience and, 12–13
 steps in, overview of, 31–41, 44–45
 as study and care planning tool, 286–287
 Taking Action step, 35–36
 vs. Tanner Clinical Judgment Model, 28–29
 use in clinical setting, 291–294
care in the community. *See* community, care in
care plan. *See* patient care plan
classroom case studies, use of Caputi Framework in, 293–294
clinical forethought, 60–61, 127–131
 defined, 130
 Managing Potential Complications, 154–158, 226–227, 290
 Predicting Potential Complications, 127–131, 226–227, 290
clinical judgment. *See also* Determining Actions to Take; Evaluating Outcomes and Thinking; Getting the Information; Making Meaning of Information; Taking Actions
 applying to performing nursing skills, 229–230
 Caputi Clinical Judgment Framework, steps in, 31–41
 comparing and contrasting three patients, student activity, 235–239
 competencies, application tips for, 56–57
 competencies, presentation of in chapters, 54–55
 competencies for, 8–10, 25, 41–44, 51

components of, overview, 25
vs. critical thinking, 5–6
defined, 5
deliberate practice and, 15–17
explaining your thinking and, 211–213, 258–259
factors influencing nurse's ability to use, 19–20
Learning Activity, 38–41
NCSBN / Next Generation NCLEX, clinical judgment measurement model, 7–10, 29–30
novice to expert theory, 25, 26–28
resilience and, 12–13
for safe patient care and improved outcomes, 10–12
steps in, 25, 28–41
Tanner Clinical Judgment Model, 28–29
Clinical Judgment Measurement Model (CJMM), NCSBN, 28, 29–30, 31. *See also* Next Generation NCLEX (NGN)
clinical manifestations
defined, 68
Identifying Signs and Symptoms, 68–73, 74, 283, 288–290
Clustering Related Information, 94–99
Caputi Framework for study of pathophysiology and medications, 289–290
relevant and irrelevant information, 111–117
cognitive guidance tools. *See also* cognitive guidance tools, advanced
Assessing Systematically and Comprehensively, 79–81
Clustering Related Information, 97–99
Collaborating with Healthcare Team Members, 134–135
Communicating, 184–185
Comparing and Contrasting, 125–126
Delegating, 180–181
Determining How to Implement the Planned Interventions, 175–176
Determining Important Information to Collect, 61–62
Determining Patient Care Needs / Healthcare Environment Issues, 139–141
Distinguishing Relevant from Irrelevant Information, 115–117
Ensuring Accurate Information, 84–85
Evaluating and Correcting Thinking, 206–207
Evaluating Data, 200–202
Identifying Assumptions, 102–105
Identifying Signs and Symptoms, 71–73
Judging How Much Ambiguity is Acceptable, 120–122
Managing Potential Complications, 156–158
Predicting Potential Complications, 130–131
Recognizing Inconsistencies, 108–110
Scanning the Environment, 65–67
Selecting Interventions, 151–153
Setting Priorities, 162–165
Teaching Others, 187–189
What would you do differently?, 217

cognitive guidance tools, advanced, 228
applying clinical judgment to performing nursing skills, 229–230
calling the physician or other provider, 252–254
community assessment / windshield survey, 273–277
comparing and contrasting three patients, student activity, 235–239
conflict resolution, 269
culture of safety, creation of, 271–272
delegating and setting priorities, 250–251
Determining nursing interventions based on signs and symptoms, 221
Effective, ineffective, or unrelated?, 220
electronic medical records, analysis of, 270
Evaluating and Correcting Thinking, 247
evaluating data, 246
explaining your thinking, table for, 258–259
medication administration, systems perspective, 264
National Patient Safety Goals, in a community setting, 267–268
overview of, 211–213
pain assessment, 223–225
patient care planning, 234, 256–257
planning safe care, 222
post-procedure care, 255
predicting and managing potential complications, 226–227
priorities, setting of, 240
relevant data on which to act, 231
safety and medication administration, 248–249
safety policies, implementation of, 265–266
SBAR form, completion of, 243–245
teaching others, 241–242
What to do when?, 219
what to do with the data, 232–233
Worse, better, or not related?, 218
cognitive processes
of Caputi Clinical Judgment Framework, 8–10
novice to expert theory, 25, 26–28
Collaborating with Healthcare Team Members, 132–135. *See also* Communicating; Delegating; Teaching Others
calling the physician or other provider, 252–254
Caputi Framework for study of pathophysiology and medications, 289–290
collaboration, defined, 132
Communicating, Caputi Clinical Judgment Framework, 182–185
calling the physician or other provider, 252–254
Caputi Framework for study of pathophysiology and medications, 290
Collaborating with Healthcare Team Members, 132–135
communicating, defined, 182
community, care in, 263
community assessment / windshield survey, 273–277
National Patient Safety Goals, in a community setting, 267–268

Comparing and Contrasting, 123–126
    Caputi Framework for study of pathophysiology and medications, 289–290
competencies. *See also* cognitive guidance tools, advanced; Determining Actions to Take; Evaluating Outcomes and Thinking; Getting the Information; Making Meaning of Information; Taking Actions
    application of, tips for, 56–57
    for clinical judgment, 41–44
    defined, 41
    explaining your thinking and, 211–213, 258–259
    practice, importance of, 55
    presentation of in chapters, 54–55
complications
    culture of safety, creation of, 271–272
    electronic medical records, analysis of, 270
    Managing Potential Complications, 154–158, 226–227, 290
    medication administration, systems perspective, 264
    medication administration and, 248–249
    National Patient Safety Goals, in a community setting, 267–268
    Predicting Potential Complications, 127–131, 226–227, 290
    safety policies, implementation of, 265–266
conflict
    Collaborating with Healthcare Team Members, 132–135
    conflict resolution, 269
content, explaining your thinking and, 211–213, 258–259
contextual (situation-based) thinking, 15
    defined, 17
    Determining Important Information to Collect, 60–61, 288–290
    use of, 17–18, 27
correcting thinking. *See* Evaluating and Correcting Thinking
critical thinking. *See also* clinical judgment
    vs. clinical judgment, 5–6
    unexpected outcomes, dealing with, 18–19
cultural practices, patient
    community assessment, 275
    plan of action, factors to consider, 148

D

data analysis. *See also* Making Meaning of Information
    advanced cognitive guidance tool, 246
    Caputi Clinical Judgment Framework, overview, 33–34
    electronic medical records, analysis of, 270
    Evaluating Data, 195–202, 246, 290
data collection. *See also* Getting the Information
    Caputi Clinical Judgment Framework, overview, 31, 32–33
    Determining Important Information to Collect, 58–62, 74, 288–290
    relevant data on which to act, 111–117, 231

debriefing
    defined, 14
    Evaluating and Correcting Thinking, 203–207
Delegating, 177–181
    advanced cognitive guidance tool, 250–251
    Caputi Framework for study of pathophysiology and medications, 290
delegating, defined, 177
deliberate practice
    clinical judgment and, 15–17
    defined, 15
demographic data
    community assessment / windshield survey, 273–277
    important information to collect, 60
    plan of action, factors to consider, 148
    SBAR form, 243, 253
Determining Actions to Take, Caputi Clinical Judgment Framework, 9–10, 34–35
    competencies for, overview, 42, 145–148
    Managing Potential Complications, 154–158, 226–227, 290
    Selecting Interventions, 149–153, 290
    self-directed thinking, putting it all together, 282–285
    Setting Priorities, 159–165, 240, 250–251, 290
    for study of pathophysiology and medications, 290
Determining How to Implement the Planned Interventions, 173–176
    Caputi Framework for study of pathophysiology and medications, 290
Determining Important Information to Collect, 58–62, 74
    Caputi Framework for study of pathophysiology and medications, 288–290
Determining Patient Care Needs / Healthcare Environment Issues, 136–141
    Caputi Framework for study of pathophysiology and medications, 289–290
Diagnosing, nursing process, 45–47
diagnostic tests
    caring for patient post-procedure, 255
    Determining Important Information to Collect, 62
    Distinguishing Relevant from Irrelevant Information, 115–117
    Ensuring Accurate Information, 84
    Identifying Signs and Symptoms, 70
Distinguishing Relevant from Irrelevant Information, 111–117
    Caputi Framework for study of pathophysiology and medications, 289–290
Do Not Resuscitate (DNR) order, 149

E

egocentric thinking, 100
electronic medical records, 270

302 Index

Ensuring Accurate Information, 82–85
    Caputi Framework for study of pathophysiology and medications, 288–290
    self-directed thinking, putting it all together, 285
environmental factors. *See also* healthcare setting
    Determining Patient Care Needs / Healthcare Environment Issues, 136–141
    Making Meaning of Information and, 33–34
    plan of action, factors to consider, 148
    Scanning the Environment, 63–67, 74, 283, 288–290
errors, in healthcare setting. *See* medical errors
ethical concerns, 148
ethnicity
    community assessment, windshield survey, 275
    plan of action, factors to consider, 148
    SBAR form, 243, 253
Evaluate Outcomes, NCLEX Clinical Judgment Measurement Model, 7, 9, 208–209. *See also* Evaluating Outcomes and Thinking
Evaluating, nursing process, 45–47
Evaluating and Correcting Thinking, 195–196, 203–207
    advanced cognitive guidance tool, 247
    Caputi Framework for study of pathophysiology and medications, 290
Evaluating Data, 195–202
    advanced cognitive guidance tool, 246
    Caputi Framework for study of pathophysiology and medications, 290
    defined, 197
Evaluating Outcomes and Thinking, Caputi Clinical Judgment Framework, 9–10, 36–37
    competencies for, overview, 42, 193–196
    Evaluating and Correcting Thinking, 195–196, 203–207, 247, 290
    Evaluating Data, 195–202, 246, 290
    for study of pathophysiology and medications, 290
evaluation data, defined, 197
explaining your thinking. *See* cognitive guidance tools, advanced

F

failure to rescue, 18, 49, 58, 129
feedback. *See* debriefing
focus, communication and, 183–185

G

gender
    Identifying Assumptions, 103, 104
    patient care plan, factors to consider, 148
    plan of action, factors to consider, 148
    SBAR form, 243, 253

Generate Solutions, NCLEX Clinical Judgment Measurement Model, 7, 9. *See also* Determining Actions to Take, Caputi Clinical Judgment Framework
Getting the Information, Caputi Clinical Judgment Framework, 9–10, 31, 32–33
    Assessing Systematically and Comprehensively, 74–81, 284
    Caputi Framework for study of pathophysiology and medications, 288–290
    clinical judgment competencies, tips for using, 56–57
    competencies for, overview, 42
    Determining Important Information to Collect, 58–62, 74
    Ensuring Accurate Information, 82–85, 285
    Identifying Signs and Symptoms, 68–73, 74, 283
    NCLEX and Next Gen NCLEX alignment, 52–53
    prioritizing actions and, 34–35
    relevant data on which to act, 231
    Scanning the Environment, 63–67, 74, 283
    self-directed thinking, putting it all together, 282–285
good decision-making, defined, 5
grey areas
    in decision making, 27
    defined, 26
    Judging How Much Ambiguity is Acceptable, 118–122

H

healthcare outcomes. *See also* complications; medical errors; quality improvement; safety
    accurate information, importance of, 84–85
    clinical judgment and, 5–6, 10–12, 20, 23–24
    communication, importance of, 183–184
    deliberate practice and, 16
    Evaluating Outcomes and Thinking, 36–37
    prioritizing actions and, 34–35
healthcare setting. *See also* environmental factors
    Caputi Framework, use in clinical setting, 291–294
    community assessment / windshield survey, 273–277
    conflict resolution in, 269
    culture of safety, creation of, 271–272
    first nursing position interviews, 295
    medication administration, systems perspective, 264
    policies and procedures of institution, 148
    safety policies, implementation of, 265–266
healthcare teams, collaboration with, 132–135
    calling the physician or other provider, 252–254
    Caputi Framework for study of pathophysiology and medications, 289–290
    Communicating, 182–185
    Delegating, 177–181, 250–251, 290
    Teaching Others, 186–189, 241–242, 290
high-level thinking, defined, 15
housing, community assessment, 273
hypothesis, defined, 159

Index

I

Identifying Assumptions, 100–105
    Caputi Framework for study of pathophysiology and medications, 289–290

Identifying Signs and Symptoms, 68–73, 74
    Caputi Framework for study of pathophysiology and medications, 288–290
    self-directed thinking, putting it all together, 283

Implementing, nursing process, 45–47

individualized patient care, 35–36. *See also* cognitive guidance tools, advanced; patient care plan
    comparing and contrasting three patients, student activity, 235–239
    competencies for, 43–44
    Determining How to Implement the Planned Interventions, 174–176
    Determining Important Information to Collect, 60–61, 74, 288–290
    Managing Potential Complications, 154–158, 226–227, 290
    planning safe care, 222
    plan of action, factors to consider, 148
    Predicting Potential Complications, 127–131, 226–227, 290

internal locus of control, 16
interprofessional teams, 132–135
interviews, first nursing position, 295
intra-professional team, 132–135
irrelevant information, 111–117
ISBAR (Identify, Situation, Background, Assessment, and Recommendation), 132–133, 184, 243–245
"it depends" thinking, 26–27

J

job descriptions
    delegation of tasks and, 179–180
    plan of action and, 148
job interviews, 295
Judging How Much Ambiguity is Acceptable, 118–122
    Caputi Framework for study of pathophysiology and medications, 289–290

L

legal concerns, 148
    delegating tasks and, 179–180
    Do Not Resuscitate (DNR) order, 149
Licensed Practical/Vocational Nurses (LPN/VN), 6
    delegation of tasks and, 179–180
licensing requirements, 6–10
long-term memory, 14

M

Making Meaning of Information, Caputi Clinical Judgment Framework, 9–10, 33–34
    Clustering Related Information, 94–99
    Collaborating with Healthcare Team Members, 132–135
    Comparing and Contrasting, 123–126
    competencies for, overview, 42
    Determining Patient Care Needs / Healthcare Environment Issues, 136–141
    Distinguishing Relevant from Irrelevant Information, 111–117
    Identifying Assumptions, 100–105
    Judging How Much Ambiguity is Acceptable, 118–122
    overview of, 89–93
    Predicting Potential Complications, 127–131, 226–227, 290
    Recognizing Inconsistencies, 106–110
    situation awareness, 92–93
    for study of pathophysiology and medications, 289–290

Managing Potential Complications, 154–158, 226–227
    Caputi Framework for study of pathophysiology and medications, 290

medical errors. *See also* cognitive guidance tools, advanced
    culture of safety, creation of, 271–272
    electronic medical records, analysis of, 270
    Evaluating and Correcting Thinking, 203–207
    Evaluating Data and error reduction, 197–202
    failure to rescue, 18
    Managing Potential Complications, 154–158, 226–227, 290
    medication administration, systems perspective, 264
    medication administration and, 248–249
    National Patient Safety Goals (NPSGs), 228
    National Patient Safety Goals, in a community setting, 267–268
    planning safe care, 222
    Predicting Potential Complications, 127–131, 226–227, 290
    safety policies, implementation of, 265–266
    Teaching Others and, 186–189, 241–242, 290
    unexpected outcomes, dealing with, 18–19

medication
    Caputi Framework for study of pathophysiology and medications, 288–290
    Distinguishing Relevant from Irrelevant Information, 115–117
    history, Determining Important Information to Collect, 61–62, 288–290
    safe administration, systems perspective of, 264
    safe administration of, 248–249

metacognition, 216
mindfulness, 12–13, 20

N

NANDA (North American Nursing Diagnosis Association), 46–47
National Council of State Boards of Nursing (NCSBN), 6–7. *See also* Next Generation NCLEX (NGN)

National Patient Safety Goals (NPSGs), 228, 267–268
NCLEX, 7–10. *See also* Next Generation NCLEX (NGN)
NCSBN Clinical Judgment Measurement Model (CJMM), 7–10, 28, 29–30, 31. *See also* Next Generation NCLEX (NGN)
Next Generation NCLEX (NGN), 7. *See also* cognitive guidance tools, advanced
    alignment with Caputi Clinical Judgment Framework, 52–53, 86–87, 90–91, 142–143, 146–147, 166–167, 170–172, 190–191, 194–196, 208–209
    Analyze Cues (*See* Making Meaning of Information)
    Caputi Framework, use in clinical setting, 291–294
    Clinical Judgment Measurement Model, 7–10, 28, 29–30, 31
    Evaluate Outcomes (*See* Evaluating Outcomes and Thinking)
    explaining your thinking, overview of, 211–213
    Generate Solutions (*See* Determining Actions to Take)
    nursing diagnosis, NANDA terminology and, 47
    preparation for, 6–10
    Prioritize Hypotheses (*See* Determining Actions to Take)
    Recognize Cues (*See* Getting the Information)
    situation-based thinking and, 27
    Take Actions (*See* Taking Actions)
NGN. *See* Next Generation NCLEX (NGN)
non-acute care settings. *See* community, care in
North American Nursing Diagnosis Association (NANDA), 46–47
novice to expert theory, 25, 26–28
nuances, defined, 124
nursing care plan. *See* patient care plan
nursing diagnosis, 46–47
nursing process
    Caputi Clinical Judgment Framework and, 45–47
    steps in, 45

O

objective data, 198

P

pain
    Assessing Systematically and Comprehensively, 79–81
    assessment, advanced cognitive guidance tool, 223–225
    defined, 79
    pain assessment tools, 223–224
parameters, for care interventions, 149–150, 199
pathophysiology, Caputi Framework for study of, 288–290
patient care plan. *See also* cognitive guidance tools, advanced; Determining Actions to Take
    advanced cognitive guidance tool for, 234, 256–257
    Caputi Framework as study and care planning tool, 286–287
    Communicating and, 182–185
    comparing and contrasting three patients, student activity, 235–239
    Determining How to Implement the Planned Interventions, 173–176
    Determining Patient Care Needs / Healthcare Environment Issues, 136–141
    Evaluating Data and plan adjustments, 197–202
    improved patient care and outcomes, thinking skills for, 10–12
    long- and short-term goals, 200
    Managing Potential complications, 154–158, 226–227, 290
    National Patient Safety Goals (NPSGs), 228
    planning safe care, 222
    plan of action, factors to consider, 148
    Predicting Potential Complications, 127–131, 226–227, 290
    relevant data on which to act, 231
patient education, 186–189
patient history / patient information
    Determining Important Information to Collect, 61–62, 74, 288–290
    Distinguishing Relevant from Irrelevant Information, 115–117
    electronic medical records, analysis of, 270
    Evaluating Data, 198–202
    Managing Potential Complications, 156–158, 226–227, 290
    plan of action, factors to consider, 148
    Predicting Potential Complications, 127–131, 226–227, 290
    relevant data on which to act, 231
patient outcomes. *See*

patient social support system, 148
physicians, guidance for calling, 252–254. *See also* team approach
Planning, nursing process, 45–47. *See also* patient care plan
policies of healthcare institution, 148. *See also* healthcare setting
    safety policies, implementation of, 265–266
post-procedure care, cognitive guidance tool, 255
potential complications
    Managing potential complications, 154–158, 226–227, 290
    medication administration and, 248–249
    Predicting Potential Complications, 127–131, 226–227, 290
practice, deliberate
    clinical judgment and, 15–17
    defined, 15
preconceived ideas and attitudes, 32
    Identifying Assumptions, 100–105, 289–290
    Scanning the Environment and, 63–67
Predicting Potential Complications, 127–131, 226–227, 290
    Caputi Framework for study of pathophysiology and medications, 289–290
pre-existing conditions
    Assessing Systematically and Comprehensively, 77, 288
    Clustering Related Information, 94
    Comparing and Contrasting, 125, 235–239
    Determining How to Implement the Planned Interventions, 175
    Distinguishing Relevant from Irrelevant Information, 113–114
    explaining your thinking, 211
    plan of action, factors to consider, 148

preventive measures, 129
priorities, setting of. *See also* Determining Actions to Take
   ABCD Prioritization Model, 162–165
   advanced cognitive guidance tool, 240, 250–251
   Determining Actions to Take, overview of, 34–35
   Determining How to Implement the Planned Interventions, 174–176
   Setting Priorities competency, 159–165
   time pressures and, 33
Prioritize Hypotheses, NCLEX Clinical Judgment Measurement Model, 7, 9. *See also* Determining Actions to Take, Caputi Clinical Judgment Framework
professional guidelines, 148
protective services, community assessment, 275

Q

quality improvement, 263
   community assessment / windshield survey, 273–277
   conflict resolution skills, 269
   culture of safety, creation of, 271–272
   electronic medical records, analysis of, 270
   medication administration, systems perspective, 264
   safety policies, implementation of, 265–266
quality of care, 263. *See also* healthcare setting
   communication and, 183–185

R

race
   community assessment, 275
   Identifying Assumptions, 101
Recognize Cues, NCLEX Clinical Judgment Measurement Model, 7, 9, 53–54
Recognizing Inconsistencies, 106–110
   Caputi Framework for study of pathophysiology and medications, 289–290
reflective thinking, 36–37
   Evaluating and Correcting Thinking, 195–196, 203–207, 247, 290
   Evaluating Data, 195–202, 246, 290
   Evaluating Outcomes and Thinking, 9–10, 36–37, 42, 193–196, 290
   reflection-IN-action, 37
   reflection-ON-action, 37
Registered Nurses (RN), 6
relevant information, 111–117
religion, plan of action and, 148
resilience. *See also* cognitive guidance tools, advanced
   clinical judgment and, 12–13
   defined, 12
   Evaluating and Correcting Thinking, 203–207
   explaining your thinking, 211–213, 258–259
RN (Registered Nurses), 6
rule-based thinking, 17–18, 26, 27, 45

Judging How Much Ambiguity is Acceptable, 118–122

S

safety. *See also* cognitive guidance tools, advanced
   Clustering Related Information, 97–99
   Communicating competencies and, 182–185
   culture of safety, creation of, 271–272
   Determining How to Implement the Planned Interventions, 174–176
   electronic medical records, analysis of, 270
   Evaluating and Correcting Thinking, 203–207
   Evaluating Data and error reduction, 197–202
   Managing Potential Complications, 154–158, 226–227, 290
   medication administration, systems perspective, 264
   medication administration and, 248–249
   National Patient Safety Goals (NPSGs), 228
   National Patient Safety Goals, in a community setting, 267–268
   planning safe care, 222
   Predicting Potential Complications, 127–131, 226–227, 290
   safety policies, implementation of, 265–266
   setting priorities and, 161–165
   Teaching Others and, 186–189, 241–242, 290
SBAR (Situation, Background, Assessment, and Recommendation) form, 243–245, 252–254
Scanning the Environment, 63–67, 74. *See also* environmental factors
   Caputi Framework for study of pathophysiology and medications, 288–290
   self-directed thinking, putting it all together, 283
Selecting Interventions, 149–153
   Caputi Framework for study of pathophysiology and medications, 290
   defined, 149
   setting of parameters, 149–150
self-assessment, 16–17. *See also* cognitive guidance tools, advanced
   Evaluating and Correcting Thinking, 203–207
   explaining your thinking, 211–213, 258–259
self-corrective thinking, 24
self-directed thinkers, 24. *See also* cognitive guidance tools, advanced
   Caputi Framework, use in clinical setting, 291–294
   Caputi Framework as study and care planning tool, 286–287
   Caputi Framework for study of pathophysiology and medications, 288–290
   controlling your own thinking, overview, 279–282
   defined, 6
   Evaluating and Correcting Thinking, 203–207
   explaining your thinking, 211–213, 258–259
   first nursing position interviews and, 295
   Getting the Information, putting it all together, 282–285
   resilience and, 12–13
   tips for becoming, 13–17
Setting Priorities, 159–165
   advanced cognitive guidance tool, 240, 250–251

Caputi Framework for study of pathophysiology and medications, 290
signs
    defined, 68
    Identifying Signs and Symptoms, 68–73, 74, 283, 288–290
simulations, use of Caputi Framework in, 293–294
situational awareness, defined, 92–93
situation-based (contextual) thinking, 15
    defined, 17
    Determining Important Information to Collect, 60–61, 288–290
    use of, 17–18, 27
sociocentric thinking, 100
spiritual beliefs, plan of action and, 148
subjective data, 198
symptoms
    defined, 68
    Identifying Signs and Symptoms, 68–73, 74, 283, 288–290

T

Take Actions, NCLEX Clinical Judgment Measurement Model, 7, 9, 42
Taking Action, Caputi Clinical Judgment Framework, 9–10, 35–36
    calling the physician or other provider, 252–254
    Collaborating with Healthcare Team Members, 132–135
    Communicating, 182–185
    competencies for, overview, 170–172
    Delegating, 177–181, 250–251, 290
    Determining How to Implement the Planned Interventions, 173–176
    priorities, setting of, 240
    for study of pathophysiology and medications, 290
    Teaching Others, 186–189, 241–242, 290
    what to do with the data, 232–233
Tanner Clinical Judgment Model, 28–29, 31
Teaching Others, 186–189
    advanced cognitive guidance tool, 241–242
    Caputi Framework for study of pathophysiology and medications, 290
team approach, 132–135
    calling the physician or other provider, 252–254
    Caputi Framework for study of pathophysiology and medications, 289–290
    Communicating and, 182–185
    Delegating, 177–181, 250–251, 290
    Teaching Others, 186–189, 241–242, 290
therapeutic communication, 183–185
time pressure
    Distinguishing Relevant from Irrelevant Information, 114
    Getting the Information step and, 33
transportation, access to, 274

U

unexpected outcomes. *See also* cognitive guidance tools, advanced
    culture of safety, creation of, 271–272
    dealing with, 18–19
    electronic medical records, analysis of, 270
    Evaluating and Correcting Thinking, 203–207
    Evaluating Data and error reduction, 197–202
    Managing Potential Complications, 154–158, 226–227, 290
    medication administration, systems perspective, 264
    medication administration and, 248–249
    National Patient Safety Goals (NPSGs), 228
    National Patient Safety Goals, in a community setting, 267–268
    planning safe care, 222
    Predicting Potential Complications, 127–131, 226–227, 290
    safety policies, implementation of, 265–266

V

Vocational Nurse (VN), 6, 179–180